Decision Making in
Transvaginal Sonography

Decision Making in
Transvaginal Sonography

Sonal Panchal
MBBS MD (Radiodiagnosis) PhD
Consultant Sonography Specialist
Dr Nagori's Institute for Infertility and IVF
Ahmedabad, Gujarat, India

Chaitanya Nagori
MD (Obstetrics and Gynecology) DGO
Director
Dr Nagori's Institute for Infertility and IVF
Ahmedabad, Gujarat, India

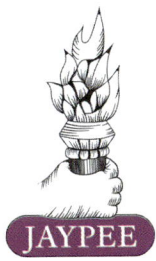

JAYPEE BROTHERS MEDICAL PUBLISHERS
The Health Sciences Publisher
New Delhi | London

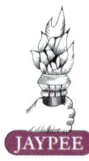 **Jaypee Brothers Medical Publishers (P) Ltd**

Headquarters

Jaypee Brothers Medical Publishers (P) Ltd
EMCA House, 23/23-B
Ansari Road, Daryaganj
New Delhi 110 002, India
Landline: +91-11-23272143, +91-11-23272703
+91-11-23282021, +91-11-23245672
Email: jaypee@jaypeebrothers.com

Corporate Office

Jaypee Brothers Medical Publishers (P) Ltd
4838/24, Ansari Road, Daryaganj
New Delhi 110 002, India
Phone: +91-11-43574357
Fax: +91-11-43574314
Email: jaypee@jaypeebrothers.com

Overseas Office

JP Medical Ltd.
83, Victoria Street, London
SW1H 0HW (UK)
Phone: +44 20 3170 8910
Fax: +44 (0)20 3008 6180
Email: info@jpmedpub.com

Website: www.jaypeebrothers.com
Website: www.jaypeedigital.com

© 2025, Jaypee Brothers Medical Publishers

The views and opinions expressed in this book are solely those of the original contributor(s)/author(s) and do not necessarily represent those of editor(s) or publisher of the book.

All rights reserved. No part of this publication may be reproduced, stored or transmitted in any form or by any means, electronic, mechanical, photocopying, recording or otherwise, without the prior permission in writing of the publishers.

All brand names and product names used in this book are trade names, service marks, trademarks or registered trademarks of their respective owners. The publisher is not associated with any product or vendor mentioned in this book.

Medical knowledge and practice change constantly. This book is designed to provide accurate, authoritative information about the subject matter in question. However, readers are advised to check the most current information available on procedures included and check information from the manufacturer of each product to be administered, to verify the recommended dose, formula, method and duration of administration, adverse effects and contraindications. It is the responsibility of the practitioner to take all appropriate safety precautions. Neither the publisher nor the author(s)/editor(s) assume any liability for any injury and/ or damage to persons or property arising from or related to use of material in this book.

This book is sold on the understanding that the publisher is not engaged in providing professional medical services. If such advice or services are required, the services of a competent medical professional should be sought.

Every effort has been made where necessary to contact holders of copyright to obtain permission to reproduce copyright material. If any have been inadvertently overlooked, the publisher will be pleased to make the necessary arrangements at the first opportunity.

Inquiries for bulk sales may be solicited at: jaypee@jaypeebrothers.com

Decision Making in Transvaginal Sonography

First Edition: **2025**

ISBN: 978-93-5696-728-1

Printed at: Sterling Graphics Pvt. Ltd. India

Preface

It was about a year back when this concept of transforming the 'transvaginal ultrasound,' a subject that requires a lot of description and essay-like presentation into short, precise, and easy-to-remember and classify, algorithm was put forward by Shri Jitendar P Vij. We do confess that for a period of 3–4 months, We kept on thinking as to how to do this conversion and whether it would be effective or not. But the persistence from Shri Jitendar P Vij's team compelled us to work on the book and to our surprise this has turned out to be a truly very precise, crisp, and a ready reckoner type of a publication. We are sure the readers will find it very useful and interesting.

Sonal Panchal
Chaitanya Nagori

Acknowledgments

With a deep sense of gratitude I thank Shri Jitendar P Vij (Group Chairman) of the M/s Jaypee Brothers Medical Publishers (P) Ltd, New Delhi, India, for the innovative concept of presentation of this book and also for pursuing me to give a proper shape to it. I also acknowledge the support of Mr Ankit Vij (Managing Director), Ms Chetna Malhotra (Senior Director—Professional Publishing, Marketing, and Business Development), Ms Pragati Singh (Development Editor), and the entire team of M/s Jaypee Brothers Medical Publishers (P) Ltd for supporting me during the preparation process of this book.

My sincere thanks to my mentor and colleague Dr Chaitanya Nagori, for his unconditional support and guidance always.

Contents

1. Essentials Before Starting a Scan 1
2. Transabdominal Scan of Pelvic Organs 2
3. Essentials of Transvaginal Scan 3
4. Doppler Ultrasound Study on Transvaginal Scan 5
5. Scan Technique for Deep-infiltrating Endometriosis 8
6. Saline Infusion Sonohysterography Procedure 10
7. Tubal Assessment by Ultrasound 11
8. Gel Vaginosonography 14
9. Transperineal Scan for Pelvic Floor 15
10. Müllerian Abnormalities 17
11. Myometrial Lesions 22
12. Benign Endometrial Lesions 28
13. Miscellaneous Uterine Lesions 34
14. Benign Cervical Pathologies 39
15. Cervical Length Assessment and Elasticity 42
16. Common Ovarian Lesions 46
17. Common Extraovarian Lesions and Pelvic Inflammatory Disease 52
18. Ultrasound in Gynecological Malignancies 57
19. Ultrasound for Diagnosis of Endometriosis 67
20. Baseline Scan 71
21. Preovulatory Assessment 76

22. **Luteal Phase Scan** 83

23. **Ultrasound Diagnosis of Polycystic Ovarian Syndrome** 86

24. **Oocyte Retrieval** 94

25. **Embryo Transfer** 99

26. **Normal and Abnormal Early Pregnancy** 102

27. **Anatomy of Pelvic Floor and Diagnosis of Descents** 114

Index *125*

Essentials Before Starting a Scan

- Detailed history of the patient related to menstrual cycles, associated pain, intercycle bleeding, obstetric history, gynecological surgeries, etc.
- Detailed history of any other nongynecological medical conditions or surgeries
- Detailed history of medicines that the patient is taking
- Set the scanner presets for Doppler [pulse repetition frequency (PRF) for color and power Doppler = 0.3 kHz, and wall motion filter at lowest, and optimal color gains)
- Set spectral Doppler sample volume as 2 mm and wall filter at 30 Hz.
- Counsel the patient and explain the procedure in detail.
- Take the consent of the patient.
- If the operator is a male, presence of a female attendant is essential.
- Establish rapport with the patient, and give her privacy.
- Select the optimal frequency probe.
- Cover the probe with a condom with gel inside and outside the condom.

Chapter 2

Transabdominal Scan of Pelvic Organs

- Transvaginal scan should be usually preceded by a transabdominal scan of the pelvis with a moderately full bladder.
- Place the probe on patient's abdomen with the patient in a supine position, having probe's lower margin on pubic symphysis and angulate towards the pelvic inlet to see the uterus and ovaries.
- For transabdominal scan, marker of the probe must always face the patient's cephalic end.
- The marker on the probe always correlates with the logo (star).
- Orientation of pelvic organs on an ultrasound image of a transabdominal scan is shown in **Figure 1**.
- Rock the probe right and left with the probe in the midline for a longitudinal survey of uterus.
- For the transverse section, always rotate the probe 90° anticlockwise.
- Orientation of the pelvic organs on the transverse section image of a transabdominal scan is as shown in **Figure 2**.
- Rock the probe up and down with the probe in the midline for a transverse survey of uterus.
- In case of difficult localization of the uterus, angulate the probe to see inside the pelvic inlet **(Fig. 3)**.
- Slide the probe on the right side or angulate on right side to see the right ovary and slide it on left or angulate on the left side for the left ovary.
- Both uterus and ovaries must be assessed in longitudinal and transverse sections.
- Scroll across both ovaries one after the other to evaluate for abnormalities.
- Assess ovaries and uterus for mobility eliciting sliding organ sign either by probe pressure or by pressure with hand on the abdomen.
- See for any free fluid.

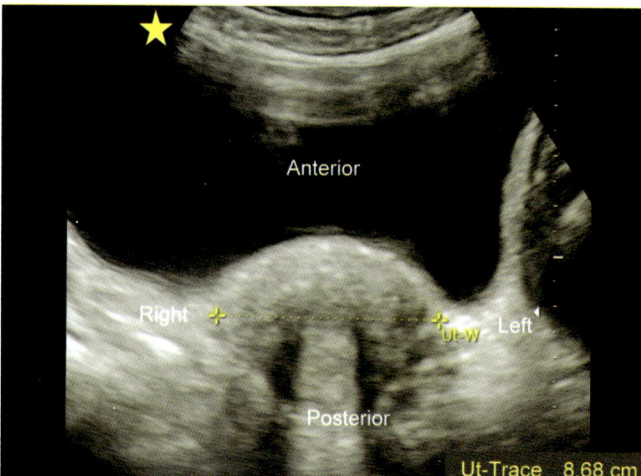

Fig. 2: Transverse section of the pelvis on transabdominal scan.

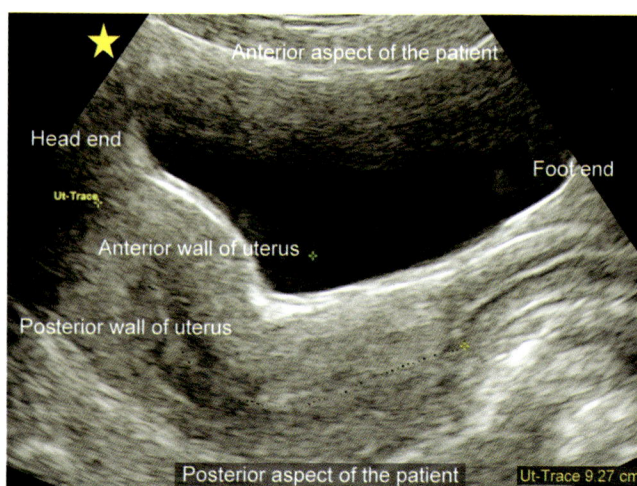

Fig. 1: Longitudinal section of the pelvis on transabdominal scan.

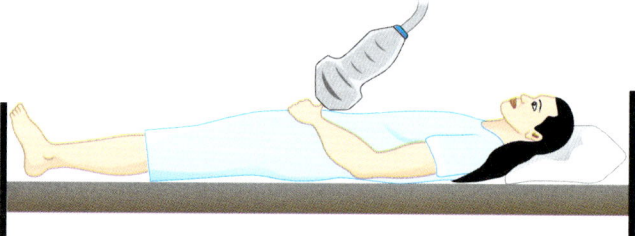

Fig. 3: Position of the probe when needed to press to localize deep-placed uterus/ovaries.

Chapter 3: Essentials of Transvaginal Scan

- Transvaginal scan is to be done on an empty bladder, in lithotomy-like position, preferably on a special couch for a transvaginal scan or gynecological couch.
- Well-lubricated probe covered with a condom or probe cover is gently allowed to slide through introitus in the vagina to see the uterus in midsagittal plane **(Fig. 1)**.
- If not seen, span the probe and midsagittal plane of uterus becomes visible, indicating deviated uterus. If part of the midsagittal plane is seen (endometrium or cervical canal), rotate the probe, this shows midsagittal plane, indicating twisted uterus.
- From the midsagittal plane, span the probe on both sides, maintaining the probe axis, to observe serosa, myometrium, endometrial–myometrial junction, and endometrium.
- Come back to the center, bring the fundus at the center of the image, and rotate the probe 90° anticlockwise to see the transverse section of the uterus **(Figs. 2A and B)**.

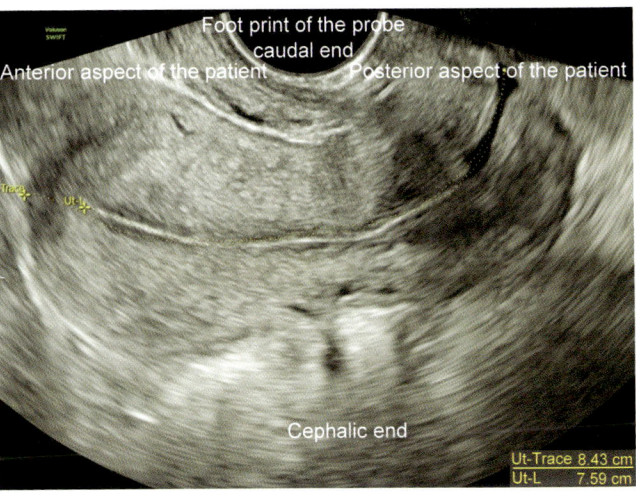

Fig. 1: Midsagittal plane of the uterus on transvaginal scan.

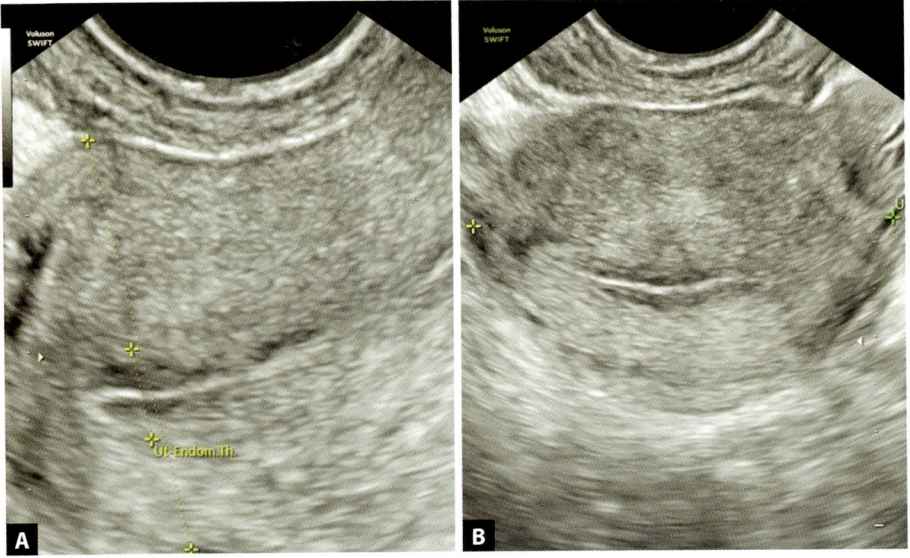

Figs. 2A and B: (A) 2D image of transvaginal scan with the uterus in midsagittal plane with fundus at the center of the image; (B) Transverse section of the uterus achieved by only 90° anticlockwise rotation from the figure A.

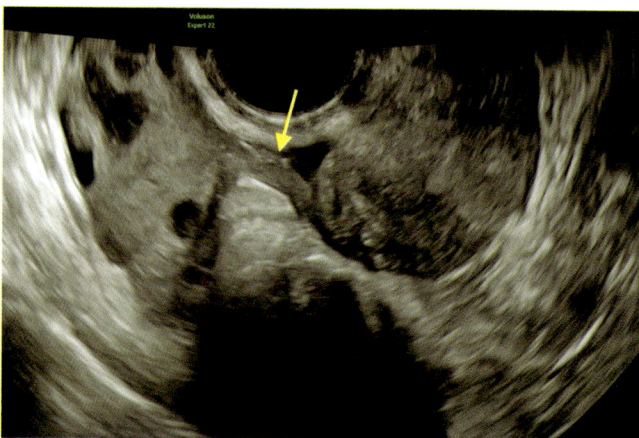

Fig. 3: Transverse section of pelvis on transvaginal scan showing uterus on right side, right ovary on the left of the image, and the yellow arrow showing soft tissue adnexal band.

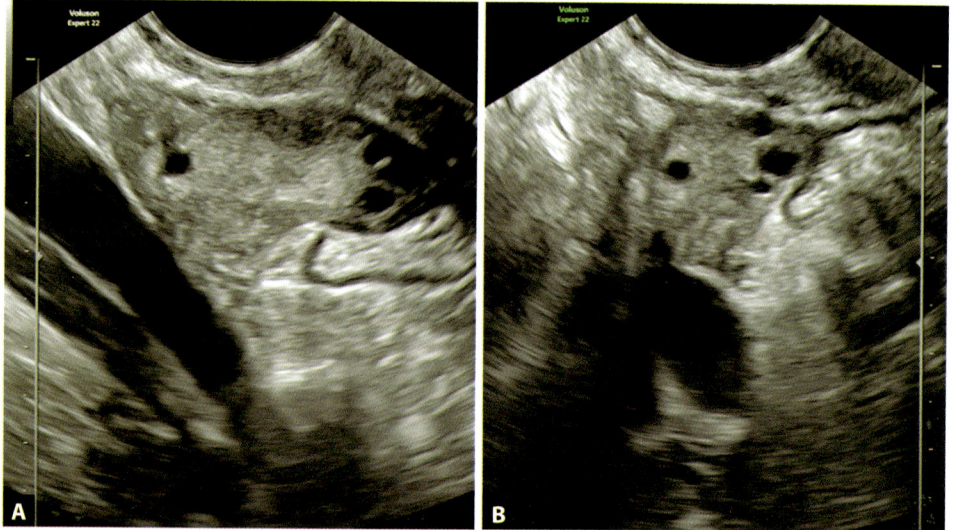

Figs. 4A and B: (A) Two long tubular anechoic structures—external iliac vessels with ovary in a long section; (B) Transverse section of ovary.

- Angulate the probe up and down to evaluate the uterus and cervix in the transverse plane.
- Come back to the fundus transverse section and span the probe following the soft-tissue adnexal band **(Fig. 3)** on any one side to follow it to ovary, if ovary is not seen just beside the uterus. If ovary is not seen there, probe is spanned to lateral pelvic wall and rotated for the transverse section of uterus. This will show external iliac vessels in long axis **(Figs. 4A and B)**. Angulate the probe superomedially, this is ovarian fossa and ovary can be found here.
- If not, from there move medially gradually, rocking the probe absolutely anterior and absolutely posterior in a zigzag path. Displaced ovary will be found somewhere on this path, may be adherent or may have long ovarian ligament.
- Finally, assess the pouch of Douglas by angulating the probe posteriorly.
- Check the mobility of the structures to rule out adhesions by in-and-out movement of the probe against uterus fundus, cervix, ovaries, and wherever two structures or organs appear to be in close apposition.

Chapter 4: Doppler Ultrasound Study on Transvaginal Scan

UTERINE ARTERY DOPPLER

- Having scanned the uterus, manage the probe to see the midsagittal plane of the uterus.
- From this plane, only span the probe from midsagittal plane to one side maintaining the same axis, till the serpiginous anechoic tubular shadows (vessels) are seen entering the uterus in the lower half of the body. Switch on the color and continue spanning the probe laterally, following the pulsatile color flow, till the lateralmost point when the vessel (artery) and the uterine wall are seen (**Fig. 1**).
- Switch on the pulsed wave Doppler, place the sample volume (2 mm, or appropriate for the diameter of the uterine artery) on this vessel, and acquire the spectrum to quantitatively assess the flow.
- The same may be done for assessment of the uterine artery flow of the opposite side.

OVARIAN STROMAL FLOW

- Once the ovary is located, bring it to the center of the image, decrease the scanning angle, and adjust the depth to allow the ovary to fill up at least two-thirds of the image. Switch on the color Doppler and scroll across or also rotate the probe if required to find vessels in the long axis.
- Set pulse repetition frequency (PRF) at 0.3 kHz and wall motion filter at the lowest.
- Gain settings should be optimum.
- Once vessels are seen in the long axis and can be traced outside the ovary, this is considered the hilar plane (**Fig. 2**).
- Once this plane is identified, the probe is scrolled across the ovary to identify bright pulsatile color spots in the ovarian stroma, away from the hilar plane and away from the follicles (**Fig. 3**).

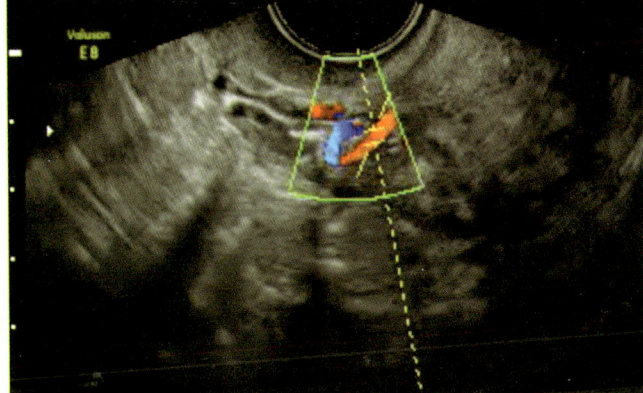

Fig. 1: Color Doppler image showing the location of the sample volume of spectral Doppler on the uterine artery on a transvaginal scan.

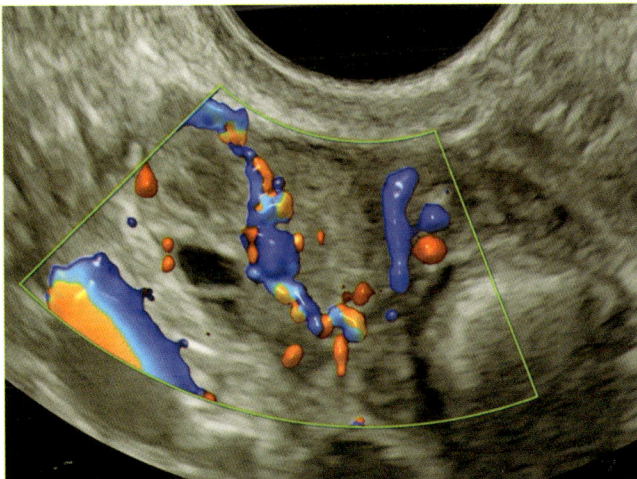

Fig. 2: Color Doppler image of the ovary on transvaginal scan showing central long vascular channel—hilar vessels, that define the hilar plane.

- Spectral Doppler assessment of the brightest of these color spots (vessels), gives the ovarian stromal flow indices.

- When there are multiple bright spots seen, the flow may be quantitatively assessed at least in three vessels and the lowest resistance index (RI) and highest peak systolic velocity (PSV) are taken as the flow indices for ovarian stromal flow.
- Angle correction is required for PSV evaluation.

PERIFOLLICULAR FLOW

- Once the ovary is located on the scan and the image is optimized so that the ovary fills two-thirds of the image, it is assessed by scrolling the probe across the entire ovary to find the grownup follicles.
- Follicle size is measured as the mean of the three longest orthogonal diameters **(Figs. 4A and B)**.
- Follicle quality is assessed by perifollicular flow.
- Switch on the Doppler and set it to cover the follicle and 5 mm of area surrounding it.
- Set PRF at 0.3 kHz and wall motion filter at the lowest.
- Gain settings should be optimum and should not be changed for consistency of results.
- Only the vessels that overlap on the follicle wall are perifollicular vessels **(Fig. 5)**.
- As color appears, gently scroll across the entire follicle to assess the abundance of the blood flow.
- Find the brightest color spots of these vessels and assess the flow by pulsed wave Doppler.
- When there are multiple bright spots seen, the flow may be quantitatively assessed at least in three vessels and the lowest RI and highest PSV are taken as the flow indices for ovarian stromal flow.
- Angle correction is required for PSV evaluation.

ENDOMETRIAL DOPPLER

- Endometrium is imaged at the center of the image in the midsagittal plane of the uterus.
- Scanning angle should be large enough to include the entire endometrium from fundal end till internal os **(Fig. 6)**.

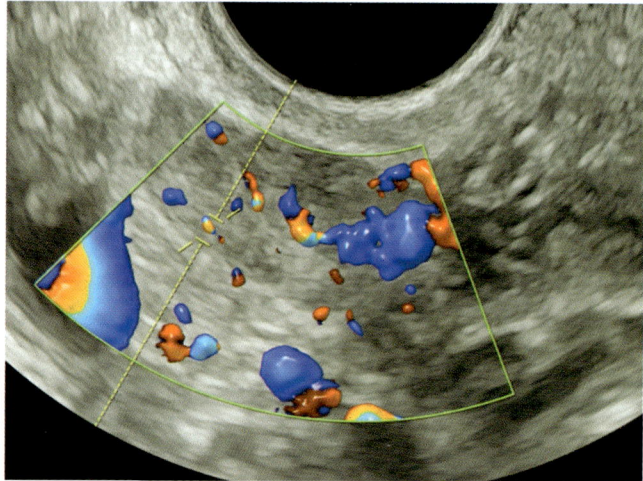

Fig. 3: Color Doppler image of the ovary on transvaginal scan showing placement of the sample volume of spectral Doppler on the stromal vessels.

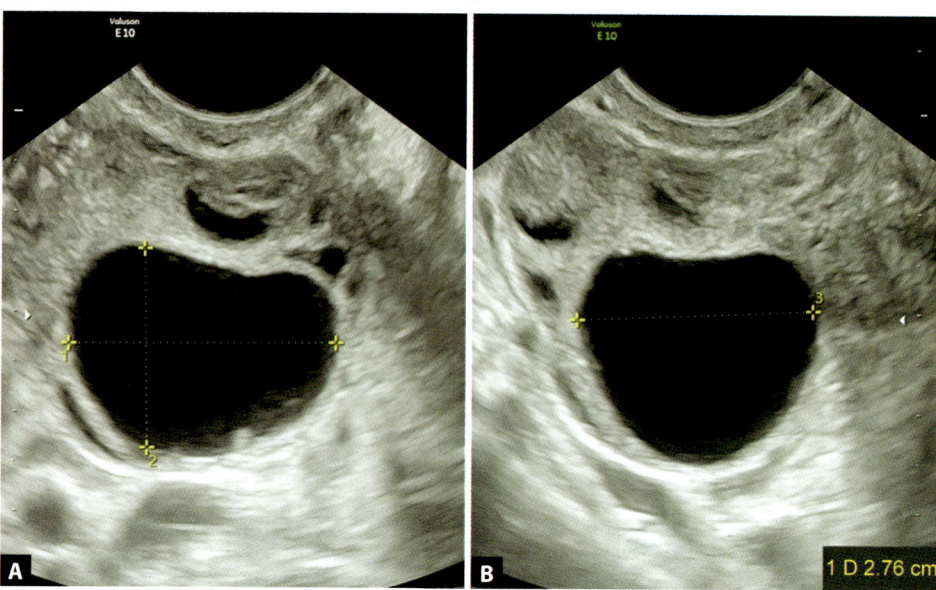

Figs. 4A and B: B-mode image of the follicle in two orthogonal planes showing measurement of three orthogonal diameters.

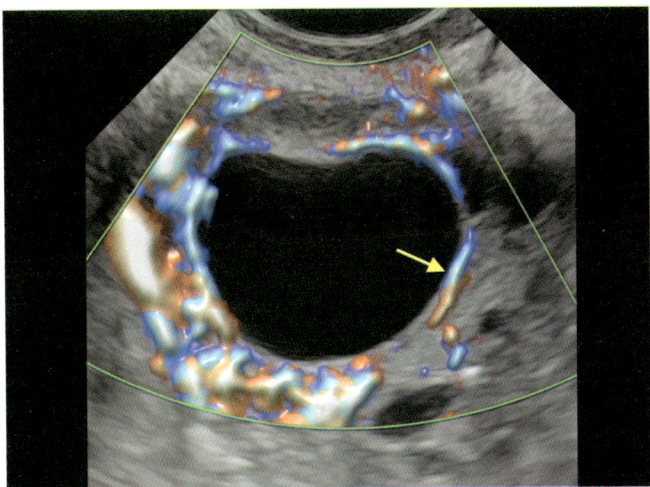

Fig. 5: Flow image showing perifollicular flow (HD).
Courtesy: Dr Sonal Panchal.

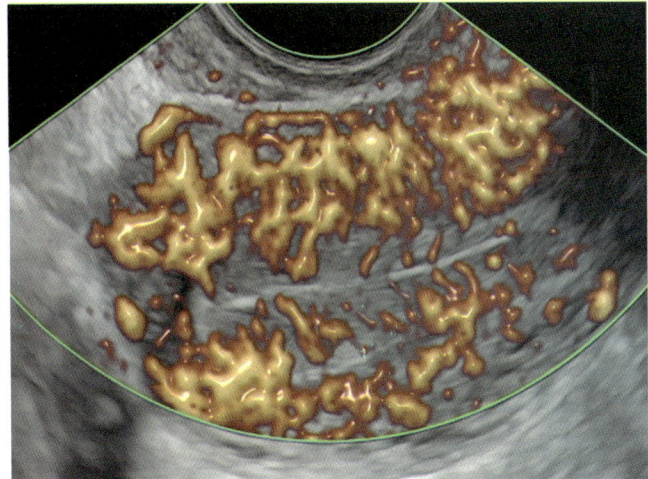

Fig. 7: Power Doppler image showing endometrial vascularity.
Courtesy: Dr Sonal Panchal.

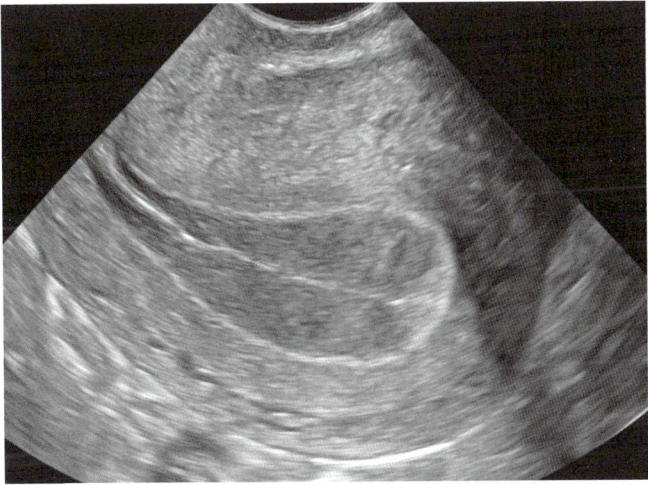

Fig. 6: B-mode transvaginal scan image of the endometrium in its midsagittal plane.

- Switch on the HD or power Doppler and place the box on the endometrium.
- The box should be large enough to include the endometrium completely and 4–5 mm on all sides beyond the margins of the endometrium.
- Set PRF at 0.3 kHz and wall motion filter at the lowest.
- Gain settings should be optimum and should not be changed from what is fixed in the preset.
- Hold the probe steadily in place for a while, it may take a few seconds for the machine to get sensitized to this low-velocity flow.
- As the flow starts showing up by Doppler, still hold the probe steady and observe the blood flow.
- All spiral vessels will not fill up in every cardiac cycle.
- Pick up an instance when maximum blood vessels are seen reaching the inner layers of the endometrium **(Fig. 7)**.
- Switch on the spectral Doppler and place the sample volume (2 mm) on the brightest vessels inside the endometrium to take a trace to quantitatively measure the flow of these vessels.

Chapter 5: Scan Technique for Deep-infiltrating Endometriosis

INTRODUCTION

Transvaginal sonography (TVS) is the first-line imaging technique in the diagnosis of pelvic endometriosis and in particular for deep-infiltrating endometriosis (DIE). Bowel preparation may improve the diagnostic ability.

Detailed history-taking and precise examination technique (to locate tender points) are important.

IMPORTANT HISTORY POINTS

- Age, height, weight, ethnic origin, and parity
- Bleeding pattern (regular, irregular, or absent)
- Last menstrual period
- Family history of endometriosis
- Previous myomectomy or cesarean delivery
- Previous surgical or nonsurgical treatment for endometriosis
- Subfertility including duration of subfertility
- Treatment for infertility and outcome
- Pain (dysmenorrhea, dyspareunia, dysuria, dyschezia, and chronic pelvic pain); hematochezia and/or hematuria with onset, severity, and duration of symptoms

PURPOSE OF ULTRASOUND

- Find lesions that can relate to symptoms.
- Assess their severity.
- Map their location for the future treatment plan.

The basic steps for ultrasound evaluation for endometriosis are given in **Box 1**.

ROUTINE EVALUATION OF UTERUS AND ADNEXA

- *For diagnosis of adenomyosis look for (Fig. 1):*
    - Position of the uterus
    - Myometrial homogeneity and symmetry
    - Cause of heterogeneity
    - Extent of heterogeneity
    - Type and score of vascularity
    - Mobility of the uterus
    - Question mark sign
- *Ovarian and adnexal assessment (Fig. 2):*
    - Cystic lesion with ground-glass echogenicity
    - Fluid–fluid level
    - Sometimes may also show hemorrhagic echogenicities

BOX 1: Basic steps for ultrasound evaluation for endometriosis.[1]

Dynamic ultrasonography		
Routine evaluation of uterus and adnexa (+ sonographic signs of adenomyosis/presence or absence of endometrioma)	First step
Evaluation of transvaginal sonographic "soft markers" (i.e., site-specific tenderness and ovarian mobility)	Second step
Assessment of status of POD using real-time ultrasound-based "sliding sign"	Third step
Assessment for DIE nodules in anterior and posterior compartments	Fourth step

(DIE: deep-infiltrating endometriosis; POD: pouch of Douglas)

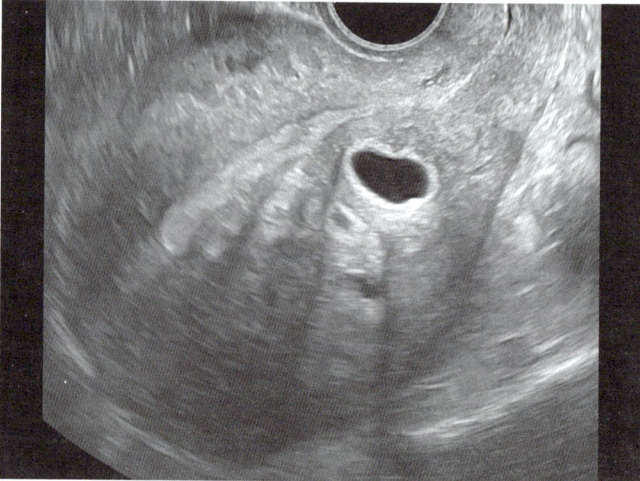

Fig. 1: Asymmetrical thickening of myometrium, hyperechoic dots and lines, myometrial cysts, fan shadows, and irregular junctional zone—signs of adenomyosis.

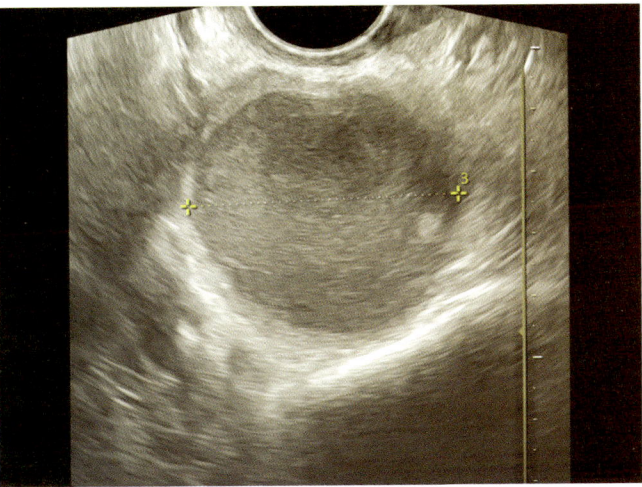

Fig. 2: Chocolate cyst with ground-glass echogenicity.

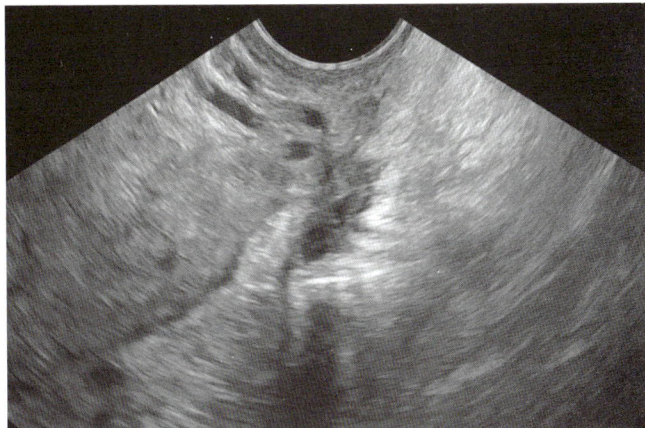

Fig. 3: Irregular hypoechoic area, interrupting the anterior muscularis of bowel with a puckered appearance and hyperechoic surrounding reaction, suggestive of bowel endometriosis.

- Hyperechoic flecks in walls
- Adhesions (soft marker)
- Kissing ovaries
- Tenderness on probe pressure (soft marker)
- Short-coursed vessels
- Associated hydrosalpinx with or without tubo-ovarian mass due to adhesions
- If there is pelvic fluid, fine strands of tissue may be seen between the ovary and uterus or the peritoneum

Assessment of Pouch of Douglas

With the sliding organ sign, elicited by in-and-out movement of the probe, establish mobility or otherwise:

- *For anteverted uterus:* Anterior rectum glides freely across the posterior aspect of the cervix and posterior vaginal wall. Ballot the uterus between the palpating hand and the transvaginal probe to see the anterior bowel glide freely over the posterior aspect of the upper uterus/fundus.
- *For retroverted uterus:* Gentle pressure is placed against the posterior upper uterine fundus with the transvaginal probe, to establish whether the anterior rectum glides freely across the posterior upper uterine fundus. Place hand over the woman's lower anterior abdominal wall in order to ballot the uterus between the palpating hand and transvaginal probe to assess whether the anterior sigmoid glides freely over the anterior lower uterine segment

Search for DIE nodules in the anterior and posterior compartments.

- *For anterior compartment:* Position the transducer in the anterior fornix and see the partially-filled bladder for any endometriotic nodules/plaques. Observe for free sliding movement between the ureter and bladder wall and anterior vaginal wall, with a free sliding movement between these layers. Also, slide the probe on both sides one by one at the level of the bladder base, to observe vesicoureteric junctions on both sides. Ureters appear as long tubular hypoechoic structures, with a thick hyperechoic mantle, extending from the lateral aspect of the bladder base towards the common iliac vessels. Scan kidneys for hydronephrosis.
- *For posterior compartment:* Pull the probe out after TVS and place it on the introitus. Then angulate it posteriorly towards the anal canal and rectum. Gently slide the probe inclining it posteriorly, tracing the interface between the posterior vaginal wall and rectum and the anterior muscularis of the anal canal and rectum. Follow it till the fundus of the uterus, which usually correlates with the sigmoid colon. Throughout the path of the probe also observe for the free sliding of the bowel on the vaginal wall to exclude adhesions. Observe for any irregularities in the muscularis of the bowel. At any such location across the path, the presence of probe tenderness is taken as guidance to locate the lesion. In case, lesion is suspected, it is evaluated on transverse section of the bowel also **(Fig. 3)**.

REFERENCE

1. Guerriero S, Condous G, van den Bosch T, Valentin L, Leone FP, Van Schoubroeck D, et al. Systematic approach to sonographic evaluation of the pelvis in women with suspected endometriosis, including terms, definitions and measurements: a consensus opinion from the International Deep Endometriosis Analysis (IDEA) group. Ultrasound Obstet Gynecol. 2016;48(3):318-32.

Chapter 6: Saline Infusion Sonohysterography Procedure

- Endometrial pathologies can often be confusing.
- Doppler and 3D ultrasound give more information than the B-mode ultrasound.
- Saline infusion sonohysterography (SIS) is the method of choice.
- First a pilot scan is done to evaluate the uterus for suspected pathologies by longitudinal and transverse sweep of the probe along the uterus.
- Probe is removed.
- Cervix is explored by per speculum (P/S) examination. The anterior lip of external os is held with tenaculum or Ellis forceps.
- Through the external os, introduce a 6 or 8 French Foley catheter to place the balloon in the cervical canal (not above the internal os). The balloon is distended only with 1–1.5 mL of distilled water or normal saline. Instead, one can also use a dedicated sonohysterography cannula **(Fig. 1)**.
- Place the probe again in the vagina, through the introitus after removing the speculum, the anterior retractor and Allis forceps, but leaving the catheter in position.
- Position the probe to see the uterus in midsagittal plane.
- Through the catheter/cannula, inject 5 mL of normal saline with the uterus seen in midsagittal plane on the ultrasound image.
- As the endometrial cavity expands with fluid, take a slow longitudinal sweep of the uterus and store.
- Rotate the probe 90° anticlockwise, with uterus still in vision. Take a slow transverse sweep and store for detailed frame-to-frame evaluation later.
- Or, one may also take a volume of the entire uterus and store as the fluid is being injected.
- After storing sufficient data, deflate the bulb, and remove the catheter.

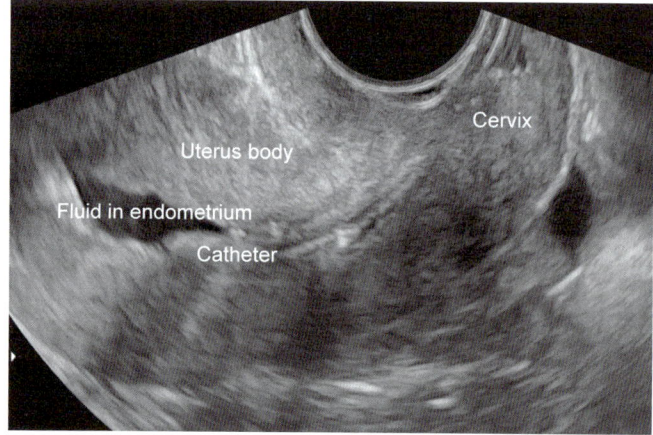

Fig. 1: B-mode image showing catheter position in the uterus.

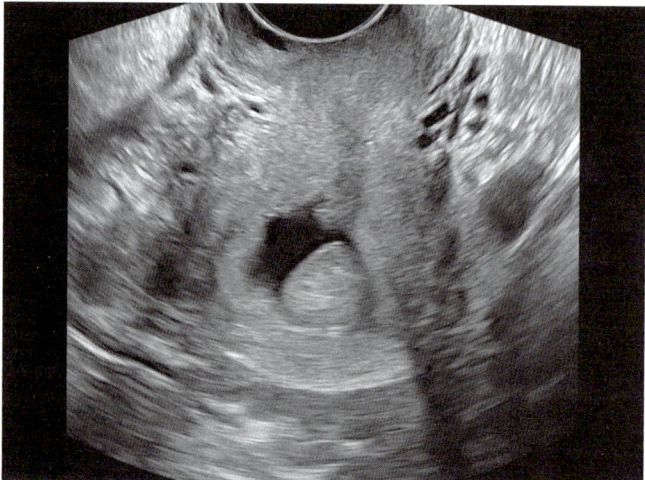

Fig. 2: B-mode image of sonohysterography showing endometrial polyp.

This is an excellent tool for the demonstration of endometrial pathologies like endometrial polyp **(Fig. 2)** and endometrial synechiae.

Chapter 7: Tubal Assessment by Ultrasound

- First, a pilot scan is done to evaluate the uterus and the ovaries for any pathologies by a longitudinal and transverse sweep of the probe along the uterus and both ovaries.
- Probe is removed.
- Cervix is explored by per speculum (P/S) examination. Anterior lip of external os is held with a tenaculum or Ellis forceps.
- Through the external os, introduce a 6 or 8 French Foley's catheter, to place the balloon just above the internal os. Instead, one can also use a dedicated sonosalpingography cannula **(Fig. 1)**.
- Balloon is distended with 1–1.5 mL of distilled water or normal saline (NS).
- Place the probe again in the vagina, through the introitus after removing the speculum, the anterior retractor, and Ellis forceps, but leaving the catheter in position.
- Position the probe to first see the midsagittal plane of the uterus to confirm the position of the Foley's balloon and then rotate the probe 90° anticlockwise to see the transverse section of the uterus **(Figs. 2A and B)**.
- Exclude any fluid collection in the pouch of Douglas.
- Then, move on to any one side at a time to be able to see the transverse section of the uterus and the ovary of that side on a single image **(Fig. 3)**.

For saline-infusion salpingography:
- Using B-mode ultrasound
- Using color Doppler
- *Using B-mode ultrasound:*
  - Through the catheter/cannula, inject 3–5 mL of NS to fill the uterine cavity and then further inject another 3–5 mL of NS slowly concentrating to see the fluid collection surrounding the ovary or trickling of the fluid from the fimbrial end of the ipsilateral tube. This confirms the patent tube **(Fig. 4)**.
  - Absence of such fluid collection may indicate a blocked tube.
  - The same procedure is repeated on the other side.
  - No fluid collection in the pouch of Douglas, distention of the endometrial cavity and complaint of pain by the patient are indirect signs to indicate bilateral blocked tubes.
  - *Limitation:* In case of unilateral block, laterality cannot be confirmed.
- *Using color Doppler:*
  - Switch on color Doppler and place the box to include the entire ovary and about 3–5 mm area surrounding it, taking care not to allow the box overlap the myometrium.

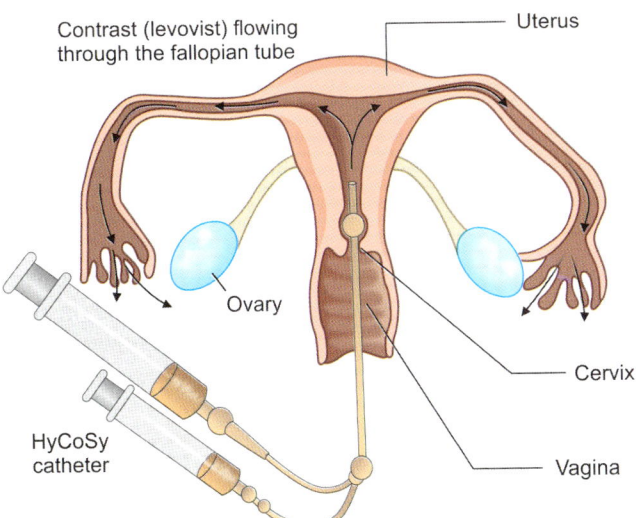

Fig. 1: Position of the balloon and catheter for evaluation of tubal patency by ultrasound.
(HyCoSy: Hystero contrast sonography)

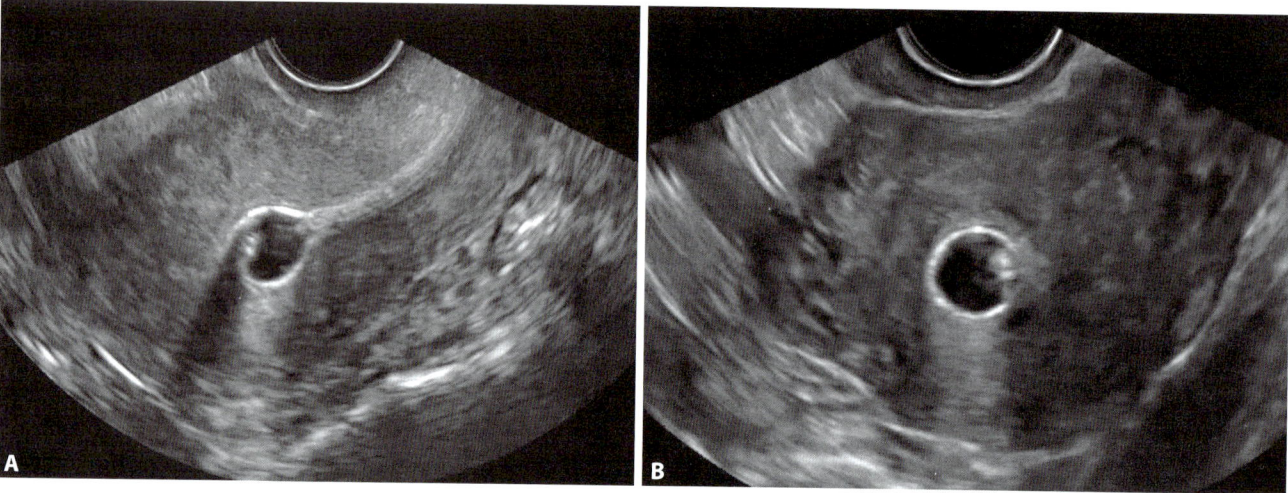

Figs. 2A and B: (A) Uterus in longitudinal section and (B) in transverse section with the Foley's bulb in position.

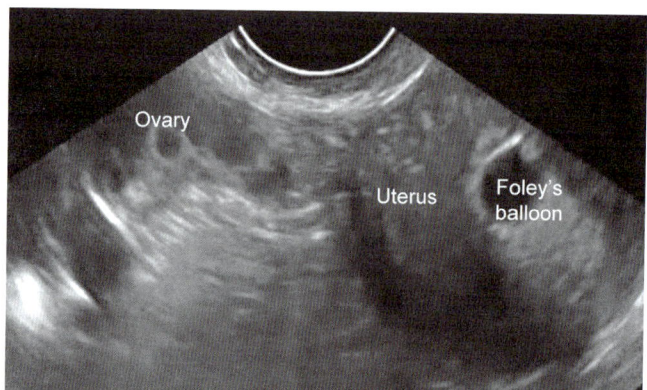

Fig. 3: 2D transvaginal scan image after Foley's insertion showing uterus and ovary in transverse section on a single image.

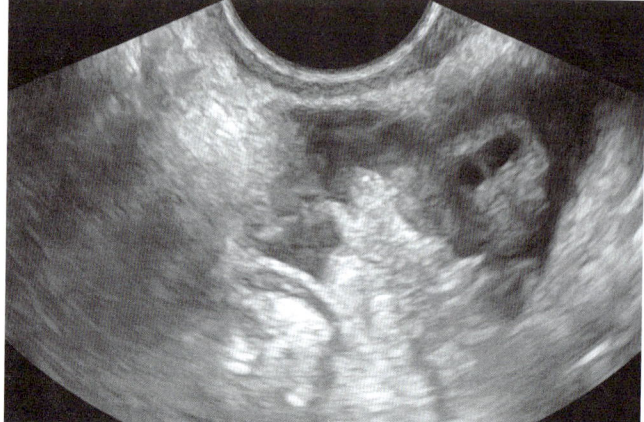

Fig. 4: Free fluid surrounding the ovary with floating fimbrial end seen on 2D image of ultrasound as a result of saline spill from the tube on saline-infusion salpingography.

- Through the catheter/cannula, inject 3–5 mL of NS to fill the uterine cavity and then further inject another 3–5 mL of NS slowly concentrating to see the color blush in the color box **(Fig. 5)**.
- Instead one may inject about 1–2 mL of NS as a short jet and observe the color blush. This has the disadvantage of causing slight pain and the patient may move, which may lead to color artifact.
- Prior instruction to the patient about the possibility of pain and request not to move may help.
- Absence of color blush indicates blocked tube.
- Same procedure is to be repeated on the other side.

For hystero contrast sonography (HyCoSy):
- HyCoSy uses positive contrast.
- The one available easily in India is "SonoVue".
- SonoVue, Bracco is sulfur hexafluoride microbubbles in NS)
- 1 mL of SonoVue is diluted with 4 mL of NS and is agitated to create foam for injection into the uterus.
- Through the catheter/cannula, start slowly injecting contrast to fill the uterine cavity and then further continue injecting, slowly concentrating to see the flow of positive contrast as hyperechoic flow beyond the interstitial part of the tube.
- This confirms patent tube.
- Contrast maybe seen outlining the entire tube and hyperechoic contrast maybe seen surrounding the ovary **(Fig. 6)**. But it may not always be seen in 2D with contrast.
- A 3D volume is acquired as contrast is being injected.
- The same procedure is done for the opposite side also.

Tubal Assessment by Ultrasound

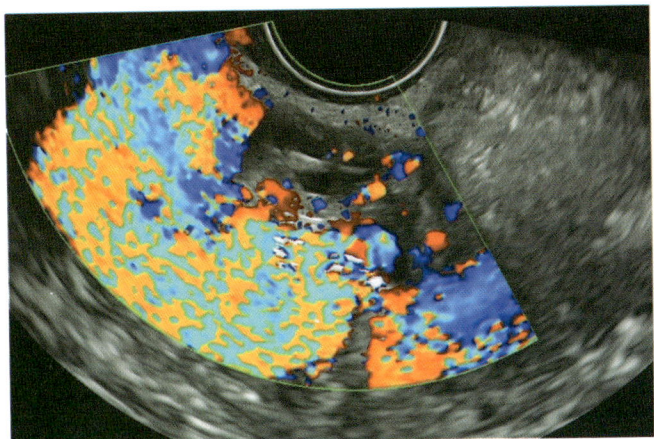

Fig. 5: Saline-infusion salpingography with color Doppler showing color blush filling up the box surrounding the ovary, suggestive of a patent tube.

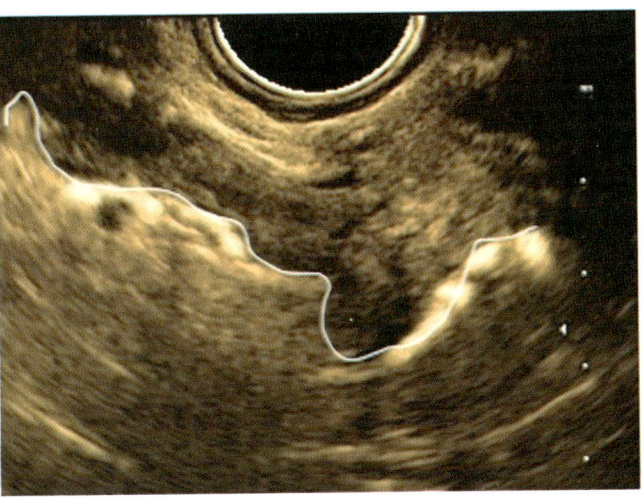

Fig. 6: Hystero contrast sonography (HyCoSy) with contrast mode—entire tube is outlined by contrast.

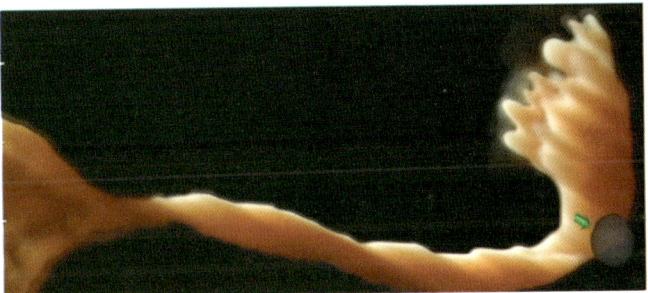

Fig. 7: 3D hystero contrast sonography (HyCoSy) with 3D reconstruction showing the entire tube with fimbrial details.

- 3D reconstruction is done on the rendered image with Magicut **(Fig. 7)**.
- That can show fimbrial details also along with tubal lumen and spill.

Chapter 8: Gel Vaginosonography

Gel vaginosonography is an investigation of choice for detailed assessment of the cervix and vagina. Though these are easily accessible clinically, their assessment with ultrasound is often inadequately done. This is chiefly so because observations of the vaginal wall and the cervix are overlooked as the probe is hastily advanced to the uterus. Moreover, since these parts are close to the probe, their detailed assessment may not be adequate with the probe used to assess the more distally placed uterus and ovaries. This can be made possible by adding a sonolucent window by the way of instilling about 20 mL of ultrasound gel in the vagina, thus allowing to place the probe far from the cervix and still allowing adequate sound beam transmission to diagnose cervical pathologies. This also may allow to study the cervical and vaginal contours, and thus identify the tissue planes and pathologies related to these. Gel may also find its way in between the tissue planes surrounding the cervix and between cervix and vagina, thus enhancing minor details. Though it does not have any major complications, it is not preferred in pregnancy and during active bleeding. Moreover, it is not recommended in every patient but is done when the following are suspected, clinically or on a transvaginal scan (TVS).

- Cervical or vaginal septa
- Cervical polyps
- Vaginal cystic lesions
- Cervical malignancies
- Vaginal endometriosis

Method:
A proper detailed TVS is done, observing the entire vaginal canal and cervix also in detail. Take off the pressure from the cervix to evaluate the cervical canal better. Take a 20 mL syringe. Take a fresh new bottle of ultrasound gel. Hold it in one hand with its mouth facing down. With the other hand, introduce the syringe nozzle into the mouth of the gel bottle and then push the outer barrel of the syringe into the bottle as the plunger is held steady. This will allow minimal air in the gel-filled syringe. Once the syringe is filled with gel, hold it horizontally in the palm, resting the barrel on the index and middle finger, and steady it with thumb and the other two fingers. Introduce the syringe into the vagina, in the posterior fornix, and introduce the gel into the vagina. Start assessing from below upward.

After the assessment of the vagina and cervix is complete, ask the patient to empty the bladder and strain out the residual gel in the vagina.

Avoiding air is the most important step in the investigation. By chance, if multiple air bubbles are introduced, the anatomical information is compromised and the procedure cannot be repeated at the same sitting.

Chapter 9: Transperineal Scan for Pelvic Floor

GENERAL SETUP

The general setup for transperineal scan includes the following:

- Patient should empty bladder prior to the scan.
- Lithotomy-like position
- Select the pelvic floor preset on a convex probe and adjust to the widest field (maximum angle).
- Place gel on the probe head and cover it with a dedicated probe cover. A glove can also be used instead to cover the probe. Gel is also placed above the probe cover. The probe is so placed on the perineum that the marker on the probe is on the anterior aspect of the patient and the margin of the probe rests on the symphysis pubis **(Figs. 1A and B)**. Volume probe may be used for 3D assessment of the perineum. 2D and volume images are acquired at rest, with full Valsalva and with coactivation.

Things to be looked for:
- Bladder volume
- Bladder wall thickness
- Bladder tumors
- Urethral diverticula
- Hematomas
- Bladder neck mobility
- Hypermobility of urethra
- Cystocele
- Cystourethrocele
- Enterocele
- Rectocele
- Rectal intussusception

Measurements to be taken:
- Extent of posteroinferior displacement of the bladder base
- Inferior displacement of the bladder neck **(Figs. 2A and B)**

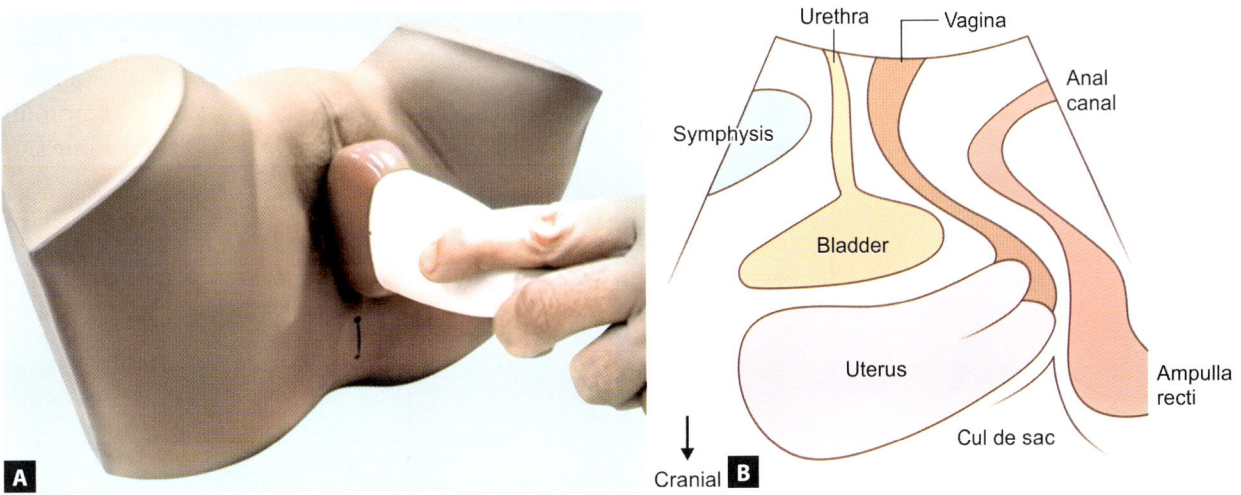

Figs. 1A and B: The position of the probe on the phantom perineum for transperineal scan.

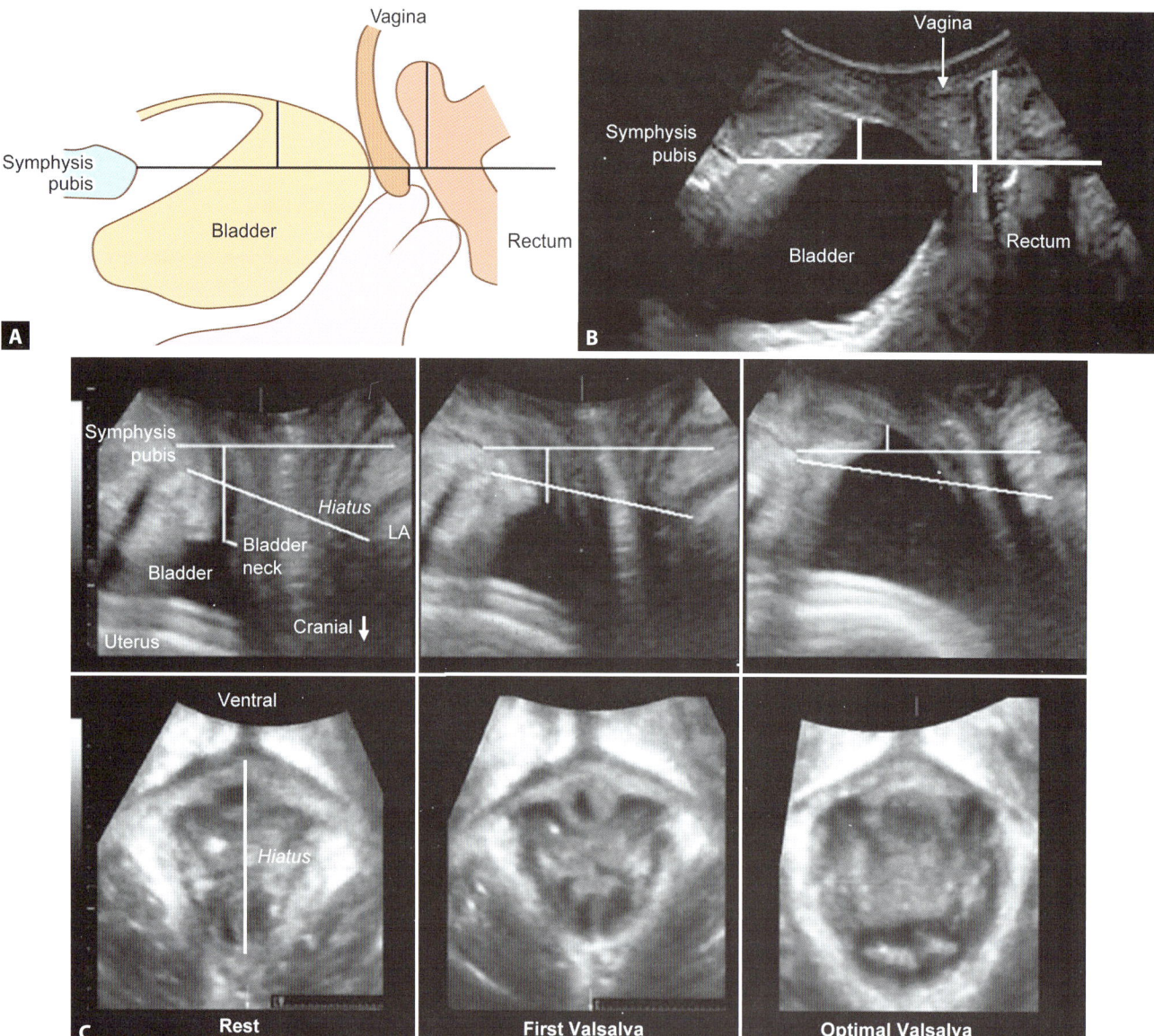

Figs. 2A to C: (A) Diagrammatic explanation of measurements to be taken for the descent of bladder; (B) The same is shown on the ultrasound image; (C) Anteroposterior and transverse diameter of pelvic outlet at rest and on Valsalva.

- Pubourethral angle
- Funneling of bladder neck
- Vesicourethral angle
- Uterine descent
- Anteroposterior and transverse diameter of the pelvic outlet at rest and on Valsalva **(Fig. 2C)**

Müllerian Abnormalities

Development of the uterus in the embryo can grossly be divided into the following steps.
- Formation of Müllerian ducts
- Fusion of Müllerian ducts
- Absorption of the intervening muscle wall

Abnormalities in the uterine shape occur depending on the time of arrest of growth during this development.
- *Formation arrest:* Agenesis of uterus and unicornuate uterus with or without rudimentary horn
- *Fusion arrest:* Bicorporeal uterus [European Society of Human Reproduction and Embryology (ESHRE)–European Society for Gynaecological Endoscopy (ESGE)] and uterus didelphys, bicornuate uterus [American Fertility Society (AFS), American Fertility Society (ASRM)]
- *Absorption arrest:* Septate uterus and arcuate uterus

There are various classifications that have been suggested for congenital uterine malformations/Müllerian abnormalities, but it needs to be understood here that Müllerian abnormalities consist of not only abnormalities of uterine body but also involve abnormalities of cervix and vagina. The old AFS classification included the abnormalities of uterus and cervix together and was probably the oversimplified form of the same. But the ESHRE-ESGE and ASRM classifications consider the uterine and cervical and vaginal abnormalities separately. The basic difference in these two classifications is that AFS/ASRM classification uses absolute measurements for assessing indentations on fundal endometrium or fundal serosa or angles between the cavities, whereas the ESHRE–ESGE classification uses myometrial wall thickness of every uterus as its own standard to assess the amplitude of deforming of serosal and endometrium. Myometrial thickness is the distance from intercornual line to the highest point on the fundal serosa, measured perpendicularly to the intercornual line. This is probably attributed to much wider knowledge of various combinations of these abnormalities. Though these are the most commonly used classification systems, congenital uterine malformations by experts (CUME) classification is also preferred by some.

ULTRASOUND DIAGNOSTIC CRITERIA

- *Agenesis of uterus* **(Flowchart 1)**:
  - Absence of dimple on the bladder base
  - No uterine shadow seen, both on transvaginal and transabdominal scan
  - Normal ovaries
  - Confirmation on MRI is essential.
- *Unicornuate uterus/hemiuterus* **(Flowchart 1)**:
  - Uterus is deviated to one side and 3D ultrasound is diagnostic, showing banana-like cavity **(Fig. 1A)**.
  - On the other side, rudimentary horn may or may not be seen.
  - Rudimentary horn is identified as an isoechoic pear-shaped structure adjacent to the ipsilateral ovary.
  - It may or may not show the central hyperechoic line of endometrium depending on whether it is functional or nonfunctional **(Fig. 1B)**.
  - It may be communicating or noncommunicating with the fully-formed horn.
  - Cervix of the fully formed horn is normal. Cervix of the rudimentary horn may or may not be formed and vagina may also have a horizontal septum. Ovaries are normal.
  - 3D ultrasound is diagnostic for uterine shape. Magnetic resonance imaging (MRI) may be required for the assessment of rudimentary horn if it is not adequately visible on ultrasound.
- *Bicorporeal/Bicornuate uterus* **(Flowchart 2)**:
  - No uterine shadow is seen in the midsagittal plane of the patient.

Müllerian Abnormalities

Flowchart 1: Algorithm for differential diagnosis of formation abnormalities of uterus.

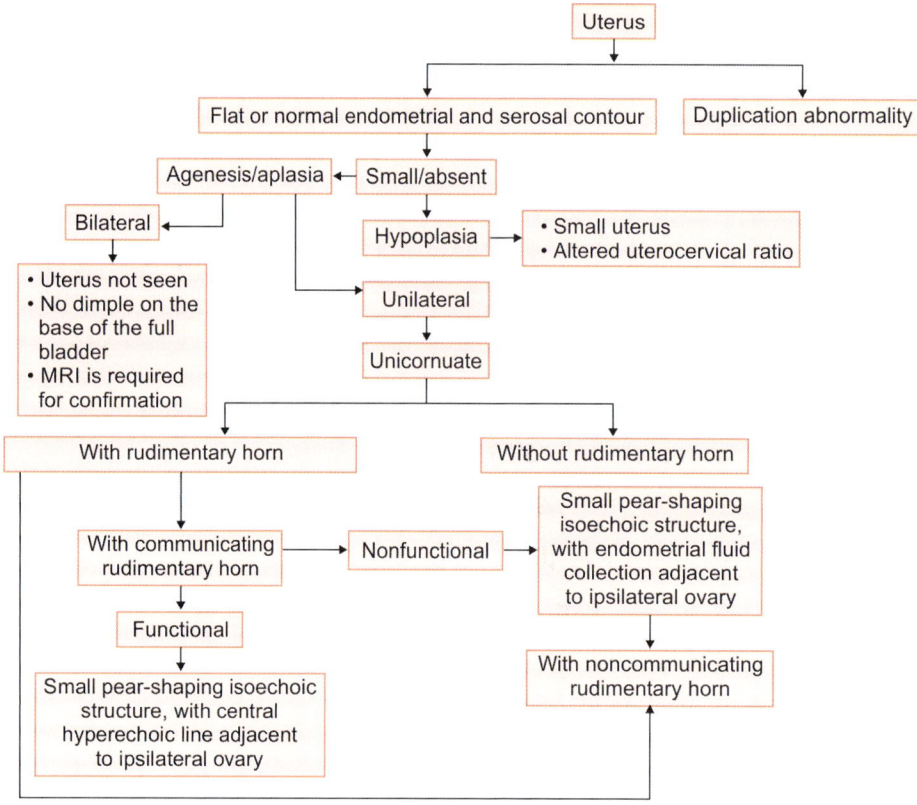

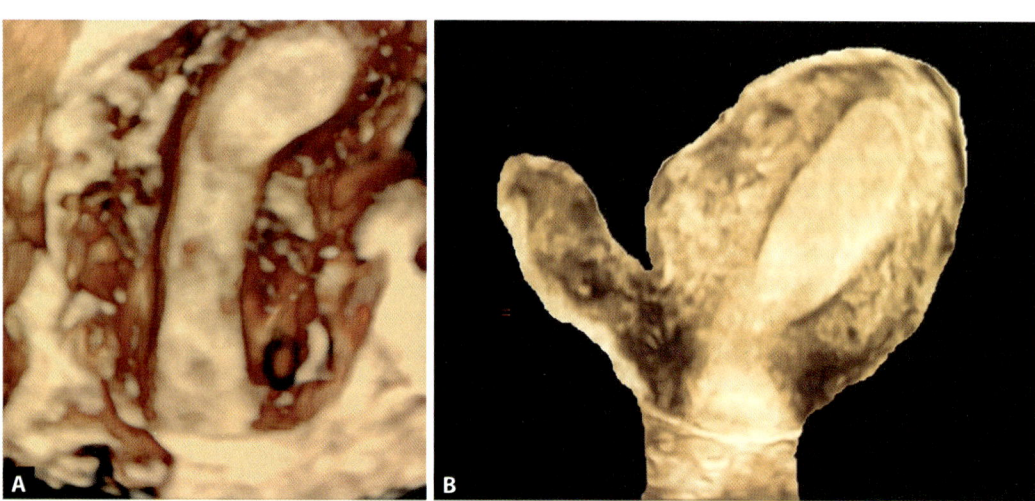

Figs. 1A and B: (A) Unicornuate uterus on 3D ultrasound; (B) 3D ultrasound image of unicornuate uterus with a rudimentary horn on right side.

- One horn of the uterus is seen on either side and pear-shaped uterine shadow one on each side **(Fig. 2A)**. Fully-formed uterine horn with central fully-formed endometrial shadow is seen on both the sides. 3D ultrasound is confirmatory as it shows a coronal view with a fundal dimple.
(*ESHRE–ESGE:* More than 50% of the myometrial wall thickness)

Flowchart 2: Algorithm for differential diagnosis of duplication abnormalities of the uterus.

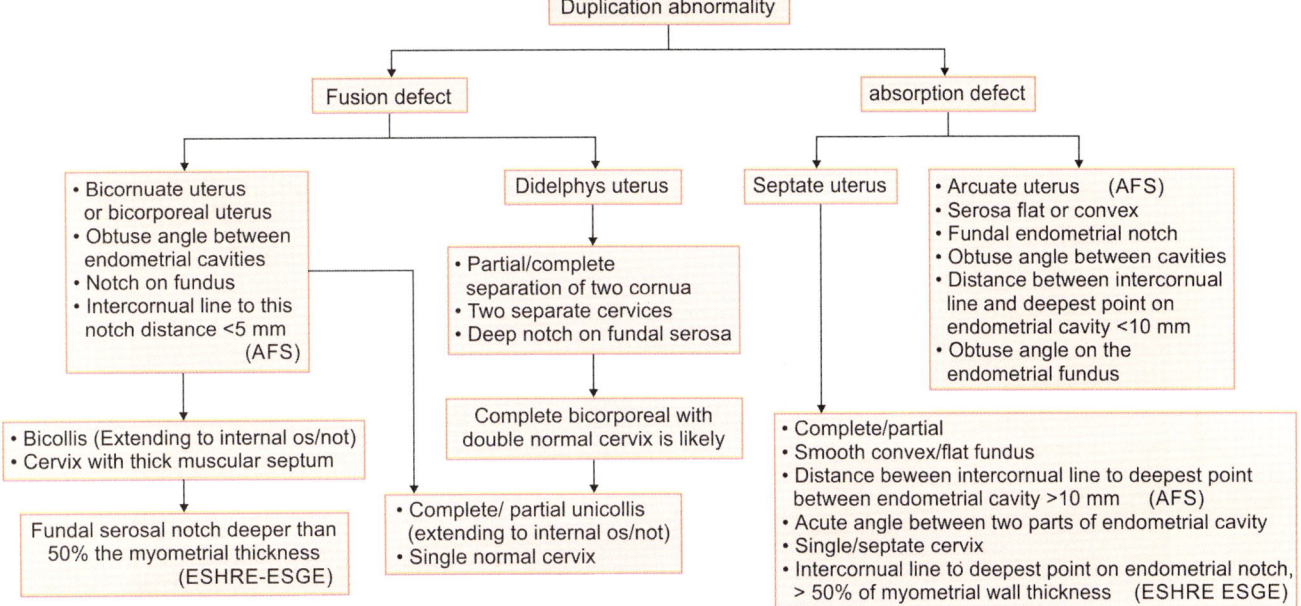

(*AFS/ASRM:* Distance between the deepest point on the notch and intercornual line of ≤5 mm, angle between the endometrial cavities of ≥105°) **(Fig. 2B)**
- Rarely the two horns may be asymmetrical. Cervix maybe single and normal (bicornuate unicollis), it maybe septated (bicornuate bicollis) or double cervix (didelphys uterus) **(Figs. 2C and D)**. It maybe complete or partial bicorporeal depending on the indentation extending to internal os or short of that. A uterus with a fundal notch and deepest point between two endometrial cavities of >1.5 times the myometrial wall thickness is "bicorporeal septate" uterus according to ESHRE–ESGE classification.
- *Septate uterus* **(Flowchart 2)**:
  - Fundal serosal shape is convex or flat. Fundal endometrium shows indentation **(Fig. 3)**.
  (*ESHRE-ESGE:* Depth of the indentation > 50% of myometrial wall thickness)
  (*AFS/ASRM:* Depth of the indentation of >10 mm and angle between endometrial cavities of ≤75°)
  (*CUME:* serosal indentation of <1 cm and endometrial indentation of >1 cm)
  - Complete or partial septum depending on the indentation extending to internal os or short of that. Septum may extend till cervix or cervix may be normal.
- *Arcuate uterus* **(Fig. 4)(Flowchart 2)**:
  - Serosal contour is convex or flat.

(*AFS/ASRM:* Endometrial indentation of <10 mm and indentation angle of >105°)
- This entity does not exist on ESHRE-ESGE classification because endometrial indentation of <50% of myometrial wall thickness is considered normal.
- Cervix is usually normal.
- *Dysmorphic uterus: (ESHRE-ESGE)***(Flowchart 1)**
  - This includes T-shaped uterus and uterus infantilis (hypoplastic).
  - T-shaped uterus is a narrow endometrial cavity due to increased lateral wall thickness **(Fig. 5)**.
  - A perpendicular is drawn from the deepest point on the lateral endometrial wall on the line joining internal os to endometrial cornu. If the length of the perpendicular beyond this line is >1.4 times the myometrial wall thickness, it is a T-shaped uterus.
  According to CUME: External angle on lateral endometrial wall of ≤130°, internal angle of the endometrial cornu ≤40°, and distance between the deepest point on the lateral endometrial wall and the *internal os to cornu line ≥7 mm*
- *Uterus infantilis (ESHRE-ESGE)/Hypoplastic uterus (AFS/ASRM)* **(Flowchart 1)**:
  - Small uterus with altered uterocervical ratio (normal is 2:1).
  - Shape of the endometrial cavity is normal.
  - Cervix is usually normal.

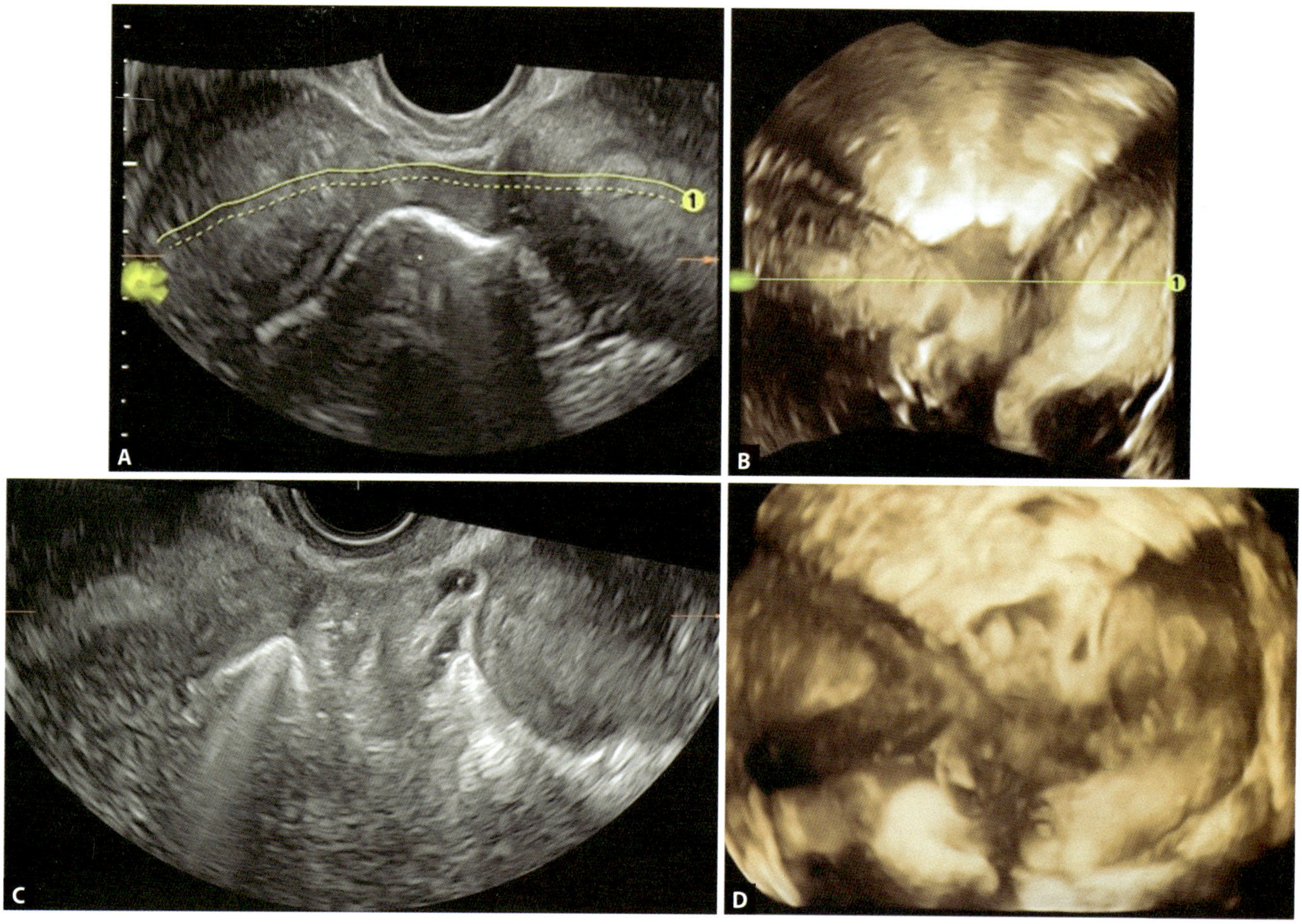

Figs. 2A to D: (A and B) Bicornuate (bicorporeal) uterus on 2D and 3D ultrasounds; (C and D) Uterus didelphys, two separate horns on 2D and 3D ultrasounds.

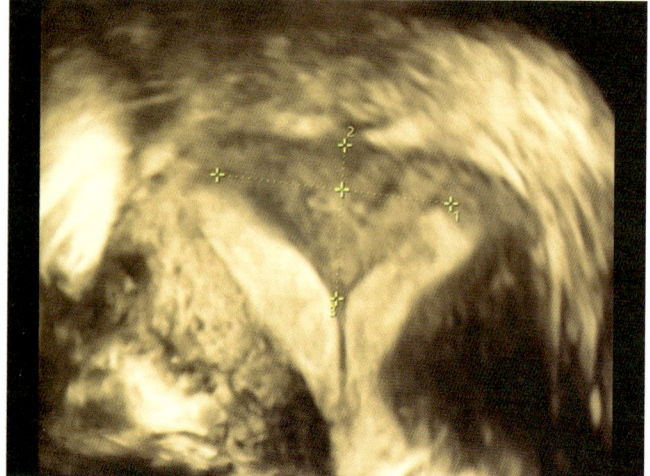

Fig. 3: Complete septate uterus on 3D ultrasound.

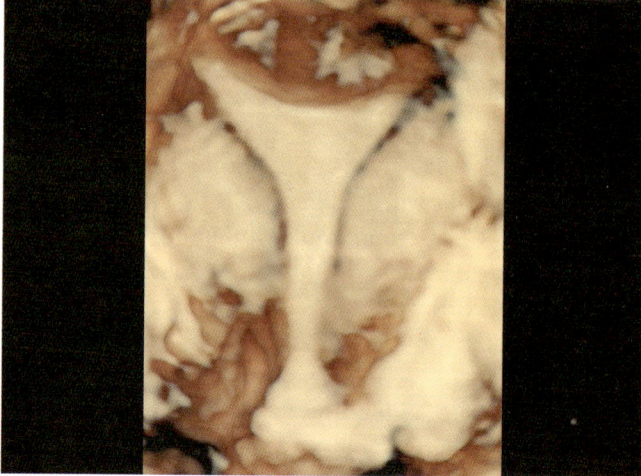

Fig. 4: Arcuate uterus on 3D ultrasound.

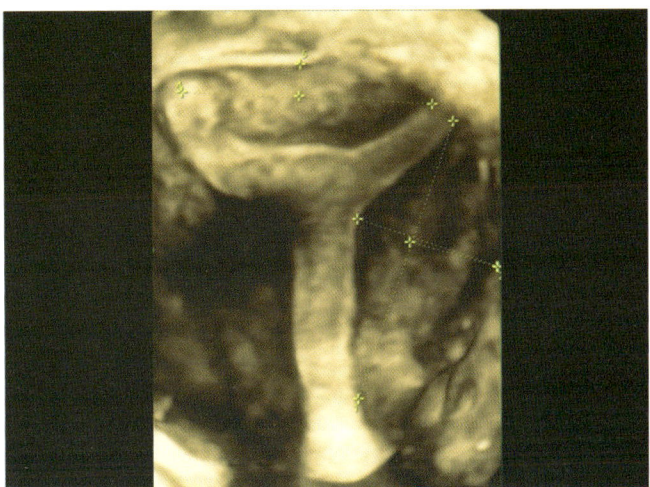

Fig. 5: T-shaped uterus.

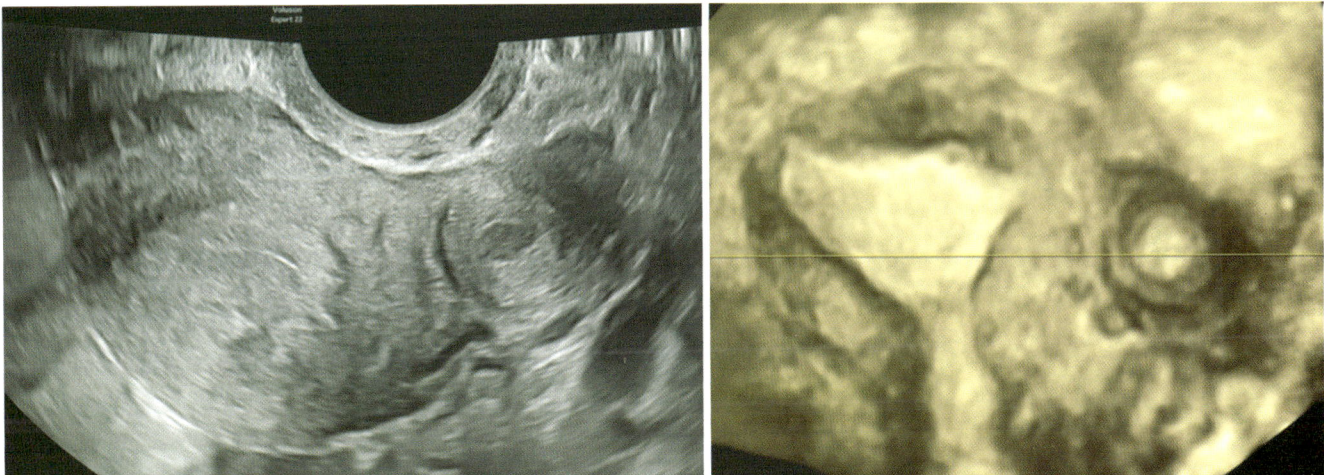

Fig. 6: B-mode and 3D ultrasound images of accessory cavitated uterine malformation (ACUM).

- Mayer–Rokitansky–Küster–Hauser syndrome is a rare congenital reproductive disorder in women, defined by an underdeveloped or nonexistent uterus and vagina.
- *Accessory cavitated uterine malformation (ACUM)* **(Fig. 6)**:
  Isolated cavitated mass, resembling a normal uterus and normal myometrium found at the level of round ligament in the presence of a normal uterus and anterolateral to this normal uterus. The cavitating mass does not communicate with the normal uterus. Ultrasound appearance is very common to that of fibroid with cystic degeneration. Patients usually present with severe pain, difficult to control with any amount of analgesics.

Myometrial Lesions

Chapter 11

An algorithm for assessment of the uterus for myometrial lesions is given in **Flowchart 1**.

ADENOMYOSIS

The imaging of uterus with adenomyosis is shown in **Figures. 1A to F**.

On B-mode:
- Symmetrical/asymmetrical enlargement of the uterus
- In case of asymmetrical involvement, details of location of the lesions are essential.
- Tenderness on probe pressure
- Heterogeneous endometrium—hyperechoic dots, hyperechoic lines, hyperechoic islands—all are due to endometrial penetration and deposits in the myometrium.

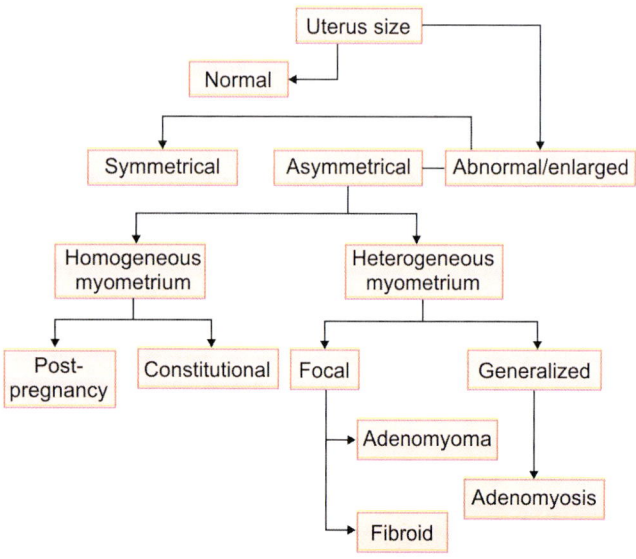

Flowchart 1: Algorithm for assessment of the uterus for myometrial lesions.

- *Anechoic myometrial cysts with peripheral hyperechoic ring:* Due to bleeding in the endometrial deposits in the myometrium and endometrial lining
- *Irregular, interrupted, or inaccessible junctional zone:* As the endometrial tissue traverses into myometrium
- In the case of hyperechoic islands and myometrial cysts, the size and location of the largest ones must be documented.
- *Fan shadows:* Alternate vertical hyper and hypoechoic shadows posterior to the lesion
- *Question mark sign of endometrium:* Reverse curvature of the endometrium toward fundus beyond the mid-body of the uterus
- Asymmetrical thinning of the endometrium

On Doppler:
- Vessels traversing the diseased myometrium, through and through, disregarding the margins
- No peripheral vascularity
- Vessels have larger diameters than normal spiral vessels.

Adenomyosis: Focal lesion

Adenomyoma and focal adenomyosis are described as follows **(Fig. 2)**:
- *Adenomyoma:* Peripheral myometrial hypertrophy that leads to fairly-defined margins
- *Focal adenomyosis:* No peripheral myometrial hypertrophy and ill-defined margins

FIBROIDS

Ultrasound evaluation of the fibroids should include:
- *Location:* Anterior or posterior, fundal, right lateral or left lateral upper, mid, or lower body or cervix
- *Size:* Three largest orthogonal diameters
- *Site/penetration:* According to International Federation of Gynecology and Obstetrics (FIGO) [PALM-COEIN (polyp; adenomyosis; leiomyoma; malignancy and

Myometrial Lesions

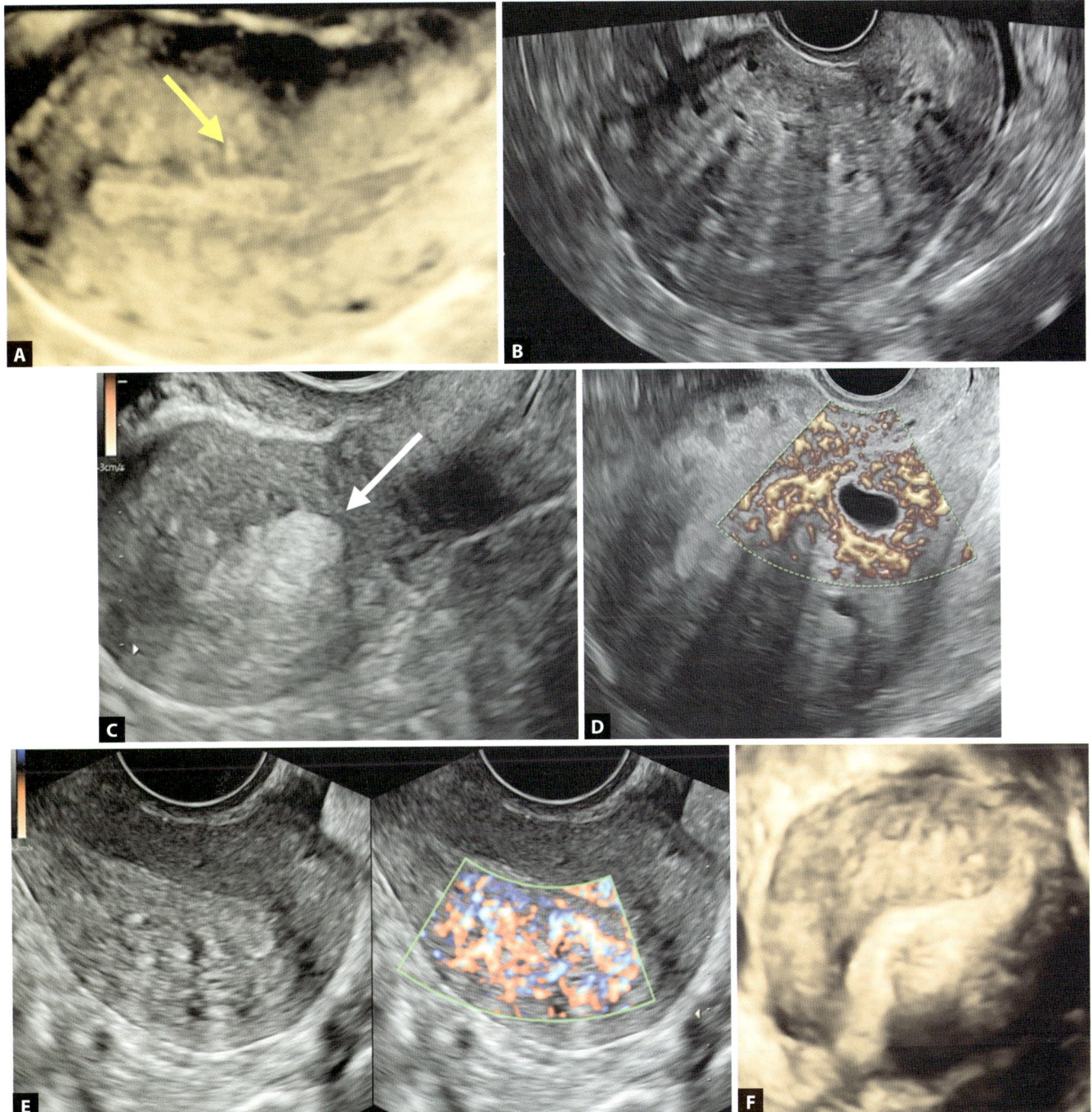

Figs. 1A to F: (A) Volume-contrast imaging (VCI) (A thick slice imaging of the sagittal section of the uterus showing irregular junctional zone (yellow arrow); (B) Thickened myometrium with heterogeneous echogenicity due to hyperechoic dots and lines with anechoic myometrial cysts and fan shadows; (C) Hyperechoic endometrial island (white arrow); (D) Fan shadows with myometrial cyst with peripheral vascularity; (E) Anterior wall adenomyosis in retroverted uterus with chaotically arranged translesional vascularity; (F) Typical question mark sign of endometrium with irregular junctional zone.

hyperplasia; coagulopathy; ovulatory dysfunction; endometrial; iatrogenic; and not yet classified) classification] **(Fig. 3)**

- Mention the *minimum distance* from endometrium *(inner lesion to free margin)* and minimum distance from serosa *(outer lesion to free margin)*

Myometrial Lesions

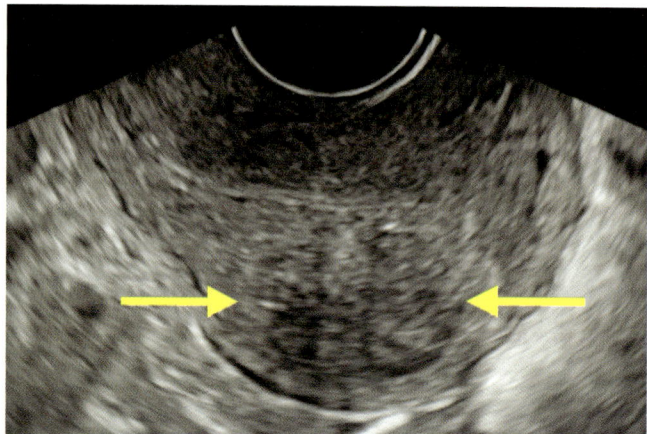

Fig. 2: Focal adenomyoma as seen between the arrows.

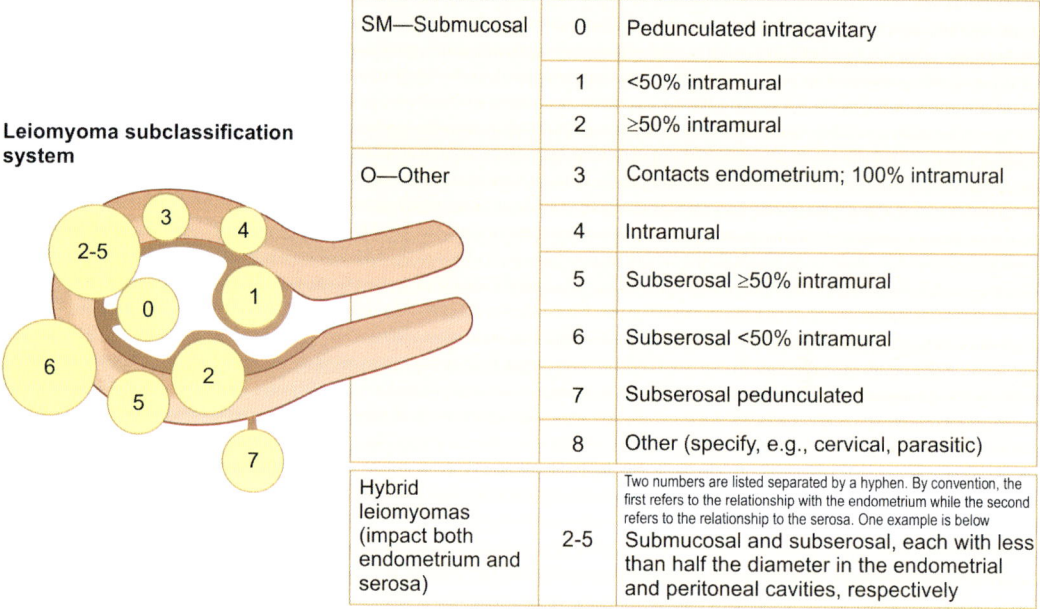

Fig. 3: Classification of localized myometrial lesions.

- *Mapping* of lesions
- *Vascularity:* Pattern, score, branching pattern, number of vessels, and diameter
- *If the lesion is present, is it relevant to the symptoms.*
- Description of the lesion:
  - Number
  - Location
  - *Echogenicity:* Homogeneous/heterogeneous
  - Hyper, hypo, or isoechoic
  - *Margins:* Well-defined/ill-defined
  - Hypo, hyper, or isoechoic margins
  - *Junctional zone:* Regular, irregular, and ill-defined
- All details of each lesion are to be documented.

On ultrasound:

- Well-defined round, oval, or lobulated solid lesion with homogeneously hypoechoic texture
- Fan shadows similar to those seen in adenomyosis are visualized but additionally a bold hypoechoic vertical shadow is seen from the lateralmost margins of the fibroid called edge shadows and is typical of fibroids.
- Junctional zone is typically regular, though in case of subendometrial (Type 0, 1, and 2) fibroids, it may be displaced **(Fig. 4)**.
- Peripheral vascularity is typical of fibroid **(Figs. 5A and B)**.

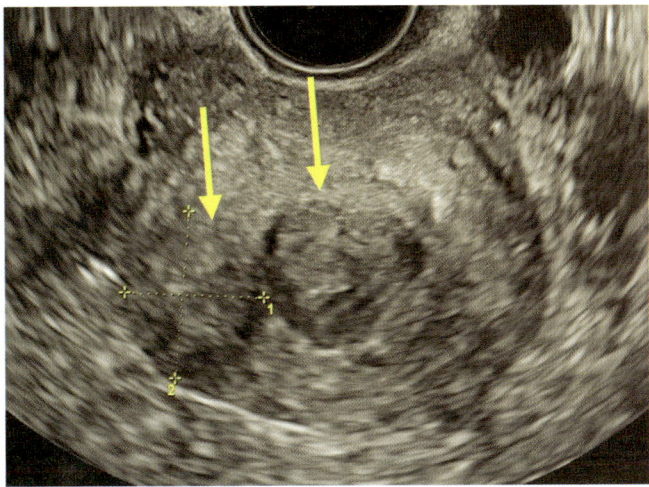

Fig. 4: Transverse section of uterus with intramural fibroid on left and intraendometrial on right (Yellow arrows).

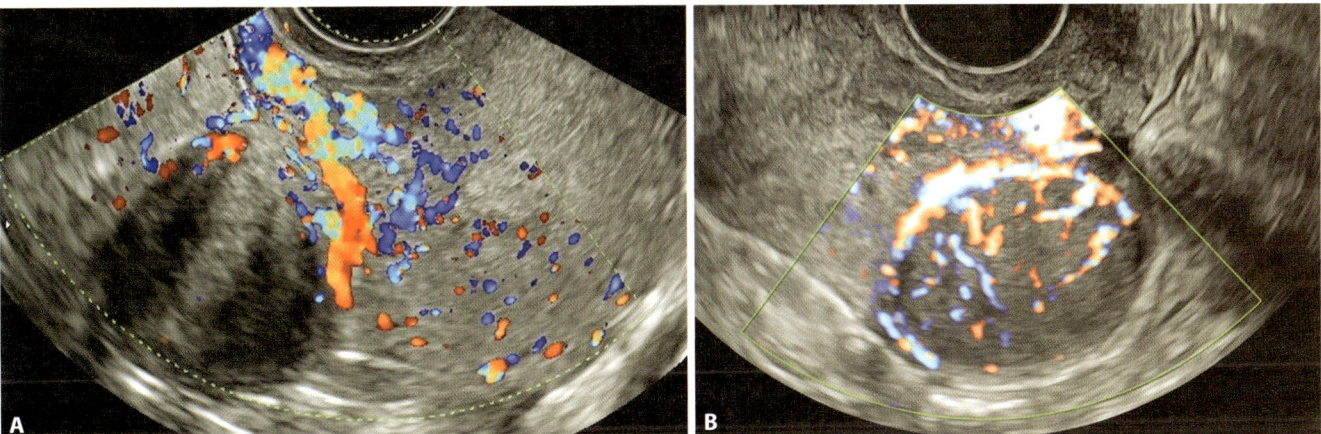

Figs. 5A and B: (A) Fibroid with peripheral vascularity on color Doppler; (B) Fibroid with peripheral and intralesional vascularity on HD flow.

- If degenerated, the fibroid shows heterogeneous echogenicity **(Figs. 6A to C)**
- There maybe hyperechogenicity, hypoechoic spots, anechoic cystic lesions, or calcifications.
- In this case, there is internal vascularity also apart from peripheral vascularity. But the internal vascularity is restricted by the peripheral vascularity. 3D ultrasound gives the best assessment of the endometrial invasion or distortion by the fibroids **(Figs. 7A and B)**.

ENHANCED MYOMETRIAL VASCULARITY

Clinical presentation:
- Heavy or irregular vaginal bleeding
- It comprises 12% of all pelvic and intraperitoneal hemorrhages and 30% require blood transfusion.[1-3]
- Maybe congenital or acquired

- Acquired may be due to previous uterine surgery, curettage, cesarean section (CS), myomectomy, endometrial or cervical carcinoma, gestational trophoblastic disease, and cesarean scar pregnancy with retained products of conception.

On ultrasound:
- Tubular, tortuous, anechoic structures seen on 2D in myometrium in a localized area **(Fig. 8)**
- On Doppler, tortuous appearing blood vessels
- If this lesion is due to retained products of conception (RPOC), products of conception may be seen in the endometrial cavity; seen on 2D and confirmed on Doppler.
- On 2D, RPOC appear hyperechoic with endometrial thickness of > 10 mm.
- Rich vascular network in the myometrium seen on Doppler with PSV of >20 cm/s (sample vol. 2 mm)

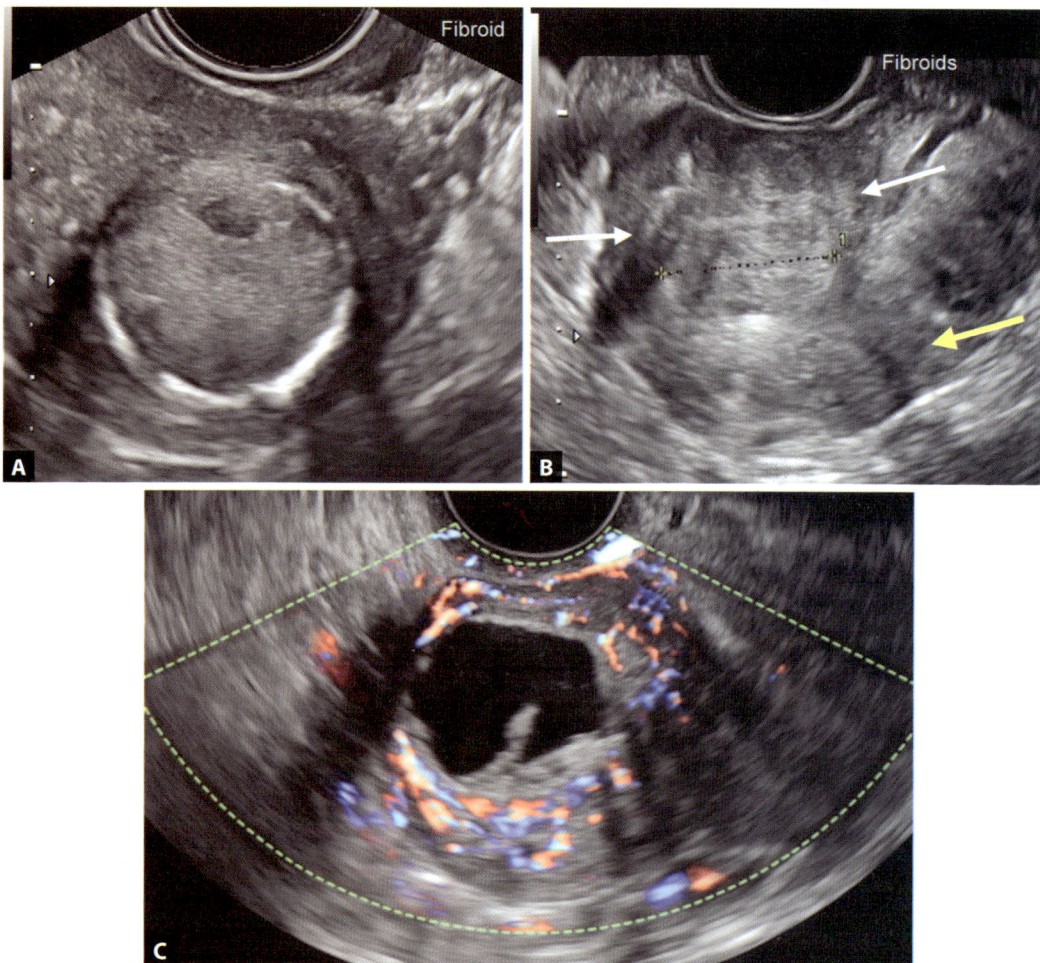

Figs. 6A to C: Degenerated fibroids. (A) Fibroid with calcified rim; (B) Degenerated fibroid with heterogeneous echogenicity; (C) Fibroid with cystic degeneration.

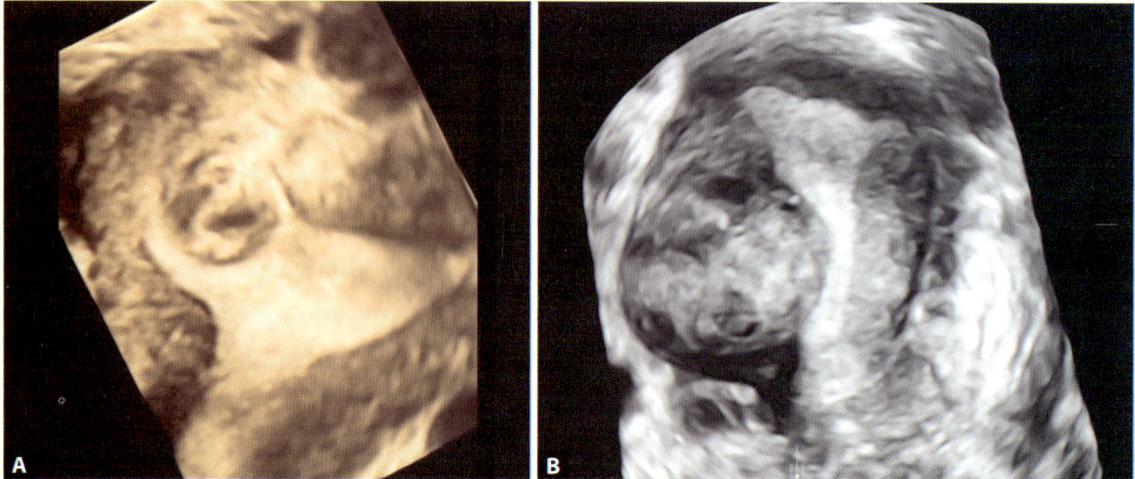

Figs. 7A and B: Cornual fibroid on 3D ultrasound; large intramural (type 2–5) fibroid distorting endometrial cavity as seen on 3D US image.

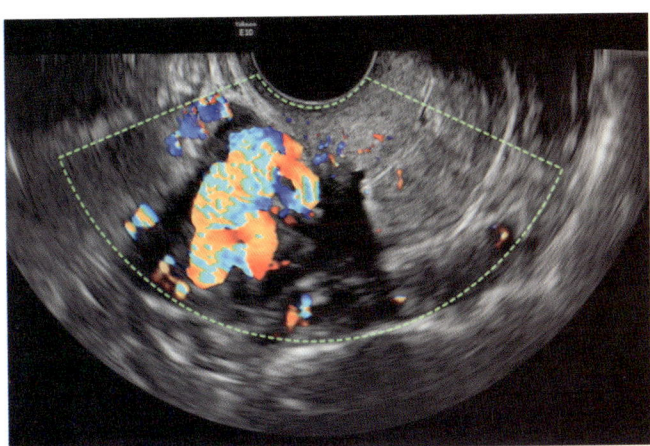

Fig. 8: Enhanced myometrial vascularity as seen on color Doppler.

(Measure the flow in multiple spots and take the maximum velocity.).
- On 3D power Doppler—knotted vessel complex
- May regress on its own
- If does not, higher risk of hemorrhage

REFERENCES

1. McIvor J, Cameron EW. Pregnancy after uterine artery embolization to control haemorrhage from gestational trophoblastic tumour. Br J Radiol 1996;69:624-9.
2. Newlands ES, Bagshawe KD, Begent RH, Rustin GJ, Holden L, Dent J. Developments in chemotherapy for medium- and high-risk patients with gestational trophoblastic tumours. BJOG 1979-84;1986(93):63-9.
3. Manolotsas T, Hurley V, Gilford E. Uterine arteriovenous malformation: A rare cause of uterine haemorrhage. Aust NZJ Obstet Gynecol. 1994; 34:197-9.

Chapter 12: Benign Endometrial Lesions

INTRODUCTION

Endometrium is the inner wall of the uterine cavity and is a receptor organ to the ovarian steroids, estrogen and progesterone, therefore it has a changing morphology and vascularity. But it also hosts certain benign lesions quite commonly. Endometrial pathologies are best evaluated in periovulatory phase of the menstrual cycle. These can be chiefly divided into inflammatory, abnormal response to hormones, and neoplastic.

PATHOLOGIES

Inflammatory

Endometrium is easily susceptible to infections because of its possibly easy access to infections through the vagina and cervix. Inflammation of the endometrium may be related to pregnancy or to pelvic inflammatory disease (PID) may it be acute or chronic **(Flowchart 1)**.

- *Acute endometritis:* Edema and hyperemia of acute inflammation lead to increased endometrial thickness with irregular junctional zone and increased vascularity and also sometimes fluid in the endometrial cavity **(Figs. 1A and B)**. Importantly, these findings should be confirmed in early proliferative phase as during the rest of the cycle, the endometrium may otherwise also be thick and hyperemic.
- *Chronic endometritis:* Chronic inflammation leads to fibrosis, and thus a persistently thin endometrium. Junctional zone is irregular and Doppler shows scanty vascularity in endometrium and subendometrium. *Synechiae* are common. These maybe identified by fluid locules in thin endometrium or saline infusion sonohysterography with 2D or 3D ultrasound (US) may be useful **(Figs. 2A and B)**.
- Tuberculosis is a common cause of chronic endometritis in developing countries. On US, tuberculous

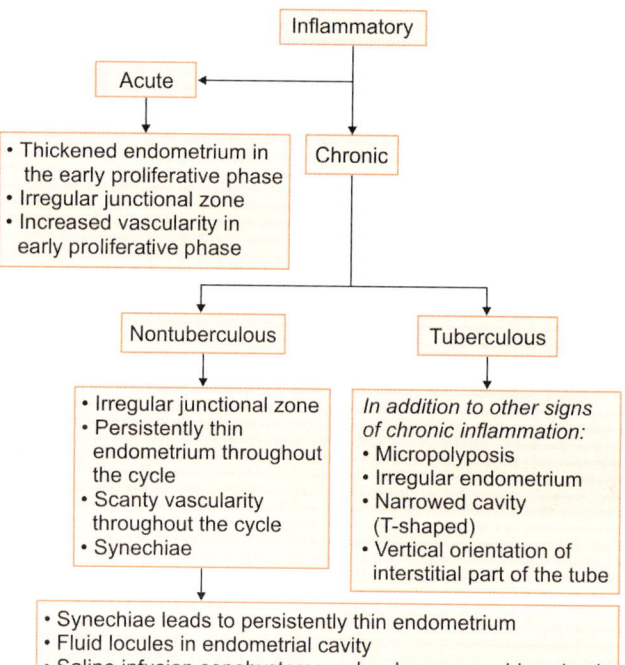

Flowchart 1: Algorithm for differential diagnosis of inflammatory endometrial lesions.

endometritis, more commonly, presents as contracted endometrial cavity, and at times as T-shaped, micropolyposis, calcifications in endometrium, junctional zone l and myometrial calcifications, fluid in endometrial cavity with hyperechoic inner walls and no flow in subendometrium, and vertical orientation of interstitial part of the fallopian tube **(Figs. 3A to D)**.

Abnormal Response to Hormones

Endometrial hyperplasia **(Figs. 4A and B) (Flowchart 2)**: Endometrium, when exposed to estrogen for a long time, leads to abnormal morphology. It appears as a thickened hyperechoic endometrium with multiple anechoic areas

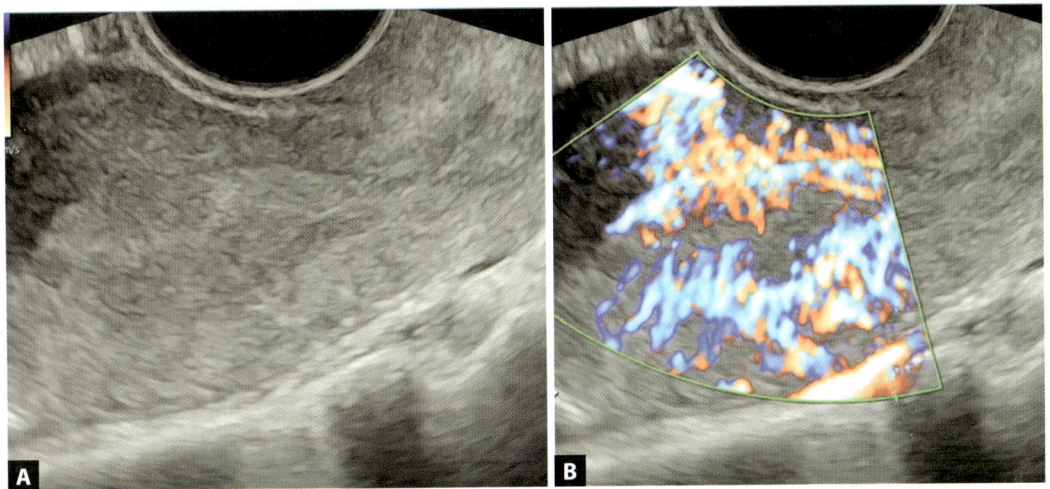

Figs. 1A and B: B-mode showing inaccessible junctional zone with thickened endometrium and increased vascularity in early proliferative phase—acute endometritis.

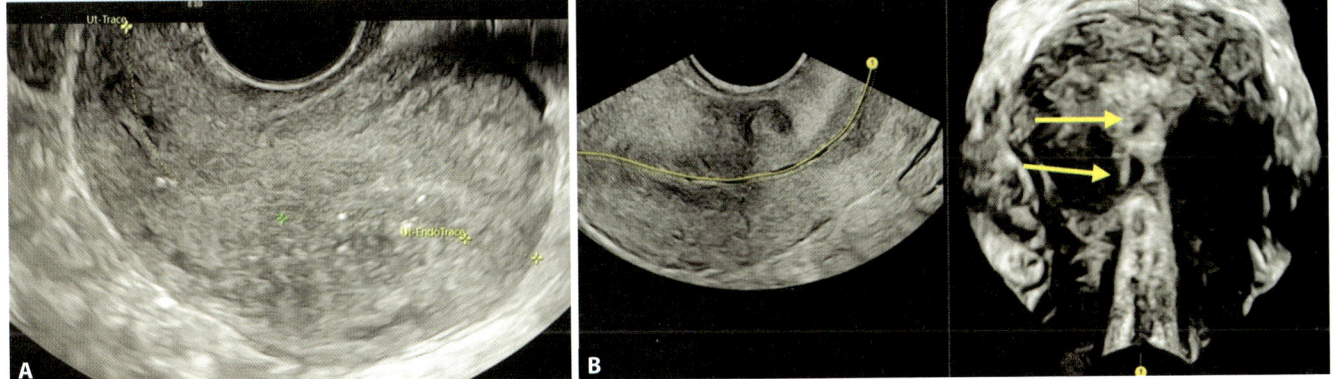

Figs. 2A and B: (A) Thin endometrium with inaccessible junctional zone and calcified flecks; (B) Thin endometrium with tiny fluid loculi (arrows) suggestive of synechiae. Both are suggestive of chronic endometritis.

and an intact junctional zone. With stromal predominance in hyperplastic endometrium, anechoic areas are tiny and almost similar in size with moderate vascularity. With glandular predominance, the anechoic areas are variable in size with some large ones and vascularity is scanty.

When a patient is on tamoxifen treatment, it has proestrogenic effect and leads to endometrial hyperplasia with a similar US image as mentioned earlier, and is called *endometrial metaplasia*. But when exposure continues for a very long time, it may result in heterogenous endometrium having blurred margins and followed by irregular junctional zone. The changes from this stage are irreversible.

Neoplastic Lesions

Flowchart 3 illustrates the algorithm for differential diagnosis of endometrial neoplastic lesions.

- *Endometrial Polyps* **(Figs. 5A to D):** These are seen as solid round or oval echogenic lesions in the endometrial cavity, visible between the endometrial lines. They are best visible in the periovulatory phase of the menstrual cycle. These may be pedunculated or sessile. Single-feeding vessel on Doppler is a diagnostic sign for polyp. These may be single or multiple and variable in size. Very large ones need to be differentiated from hyperplasia that has multiple symmetrically placed blood vessels as compared to the single feeder of polyp. Saline infusion sonohysterography may be of help with 2D US or 3D US for identification and confirmation of polyp. Polyps are common in cervix also.
- *Endometrial fibroids* **(Figs. 6A to C):** Fibroids are lesions arising from myometrium but may protrude into the endometrium and are then called

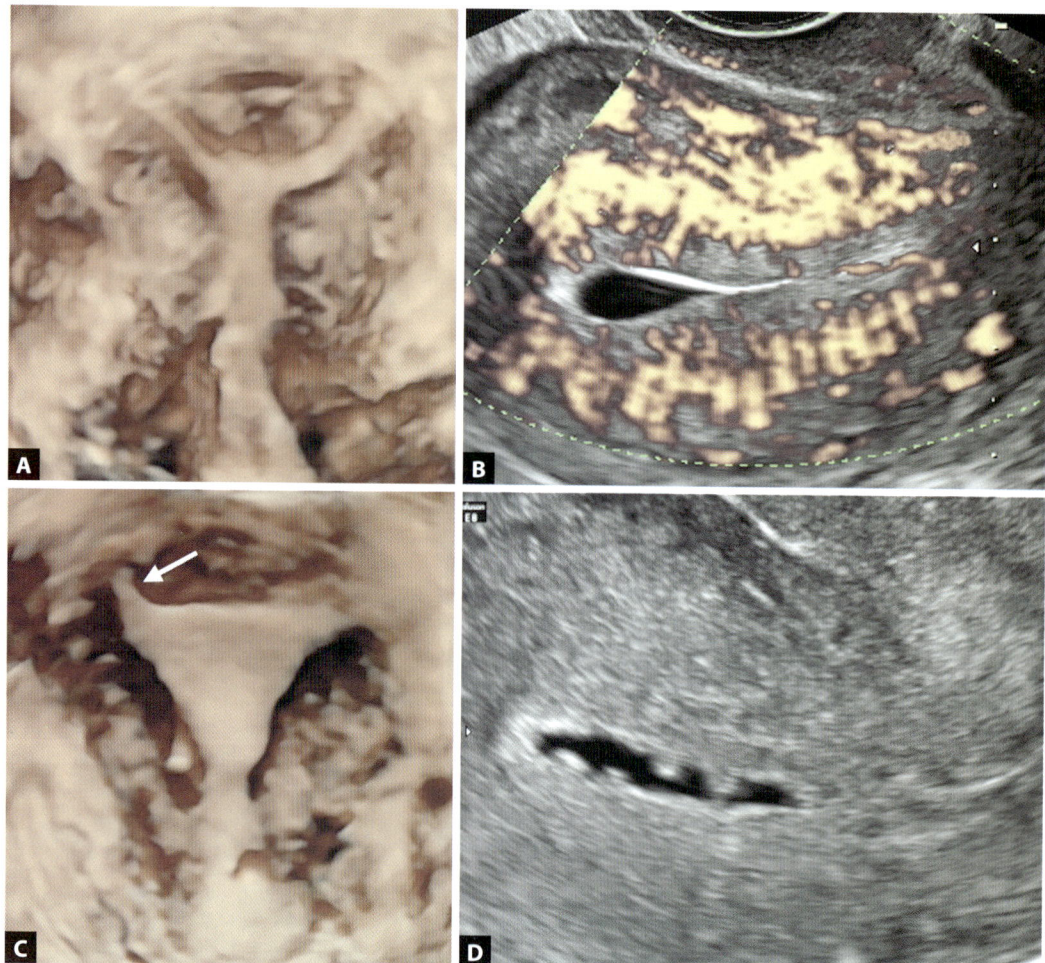

Figs. 3A to D: (A) 3D ultrasound image of the uterus showing contracted endometrial cavity; (B) B-mode and power Doppler image of the uterus in long axis showing fluid in endometrial cavity with hyperechoic inner walls and no flow in subendometrium; and (C) Vertical orientation of interstitial part of the tube (arrow) seen on 3D rendered image of uterus; (D) Micropolyposis.
Courtesy: Dr Sonal Panchal.

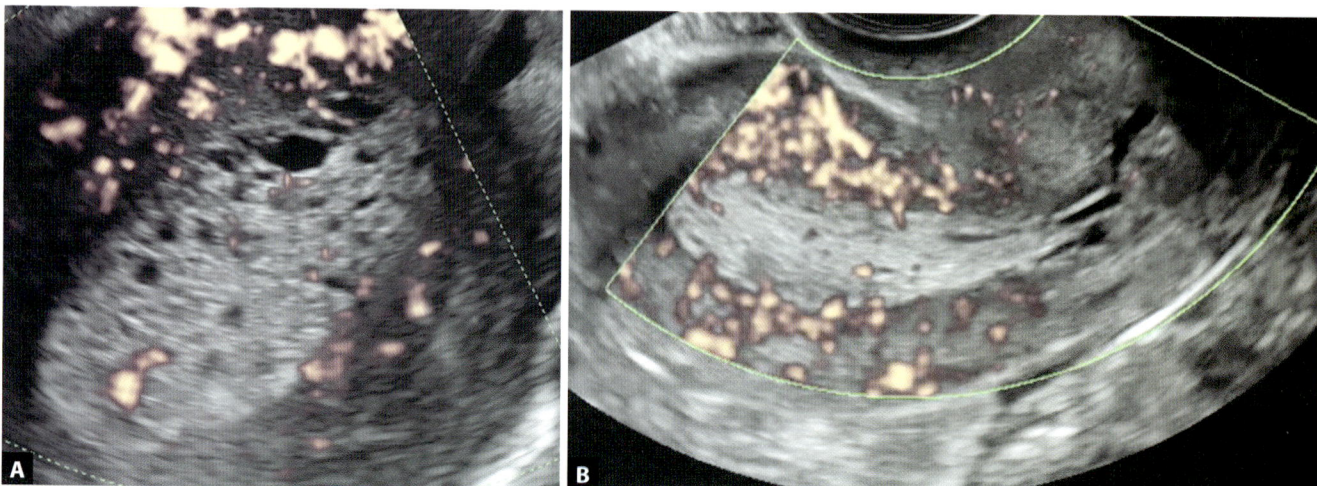

Figs. 4A and B: (A) Cystic (glandular) endometrial hyperplasia; (B) Endometrial hyperplasia with stromal predominance.

Flowchart 2: Algorithm for differential diagnosis of endometrial hyperplasia.

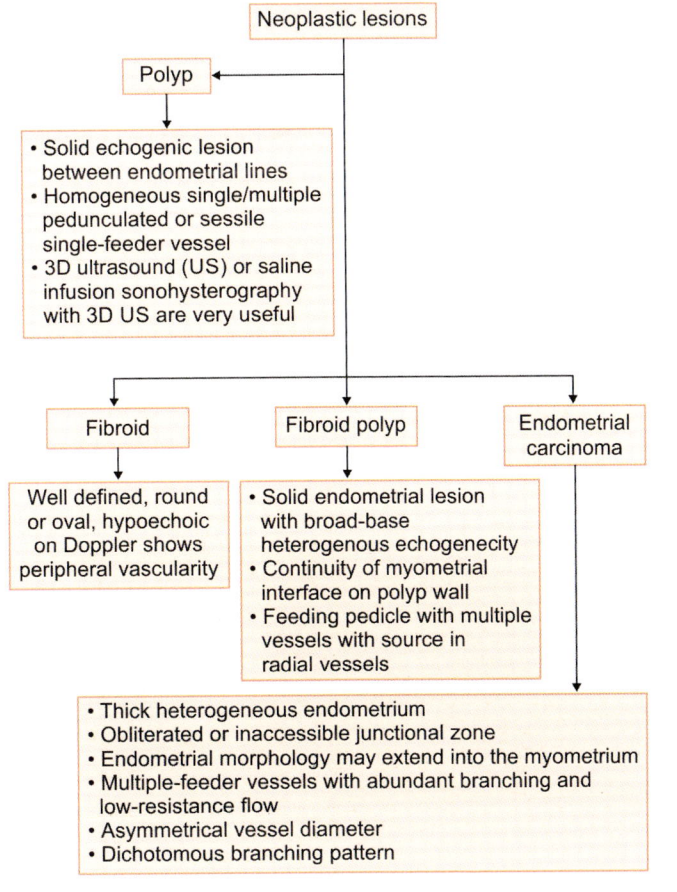

Flowchart 3: Algorithm for differential diagnosis of endometrial neoplastic lesions.

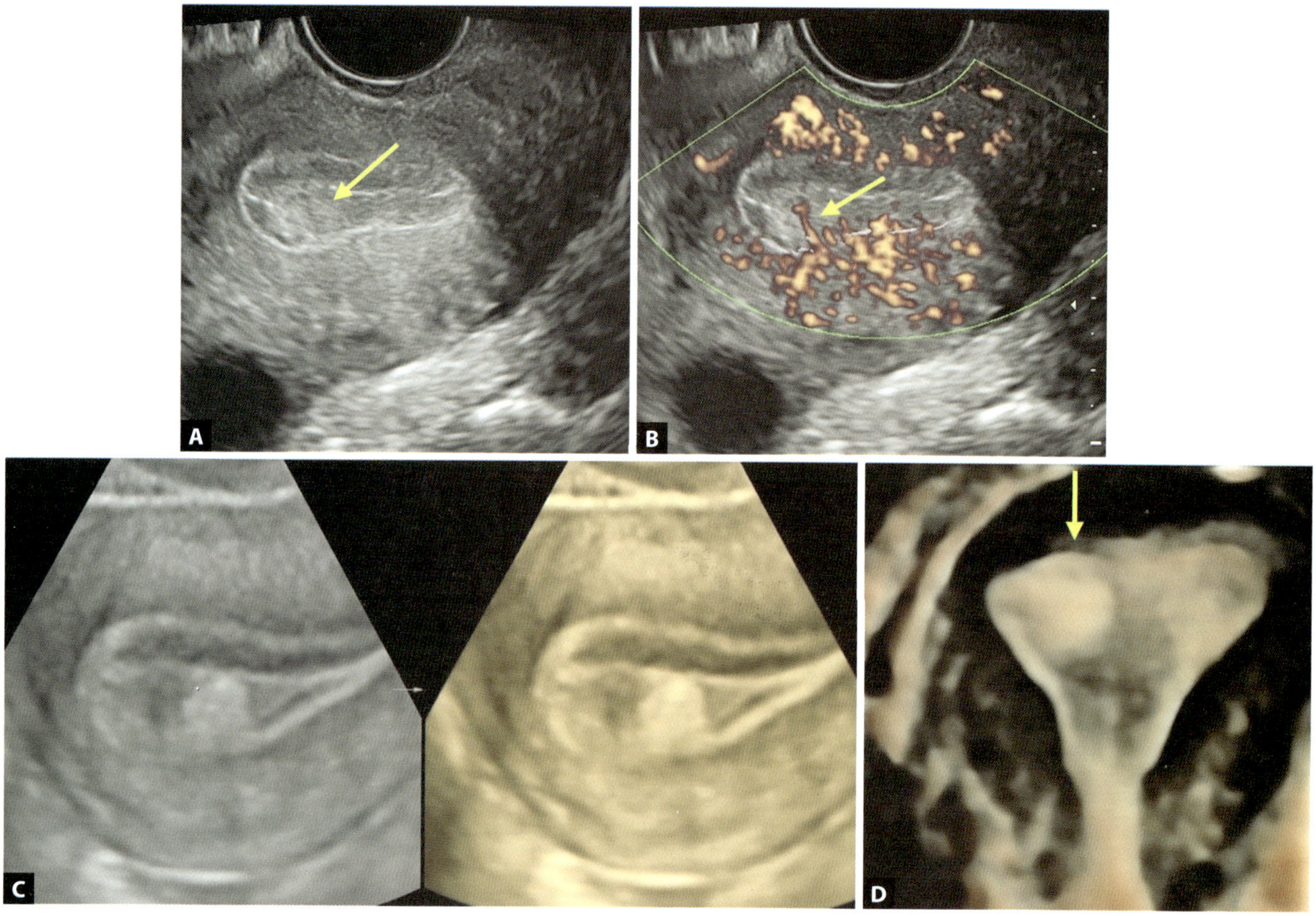

Figs. 5A to D: (A) B-mode image of endometrial polyp (yellow arrow); (B) Power Doppler image of the same showing single-feeder vessel (yellow arrow); (C) Volume contrast imaging (VCI) for better visualization of polyp with subtle echogenicity; (D) 3D ultrasound rendered image of endometrial polyp.

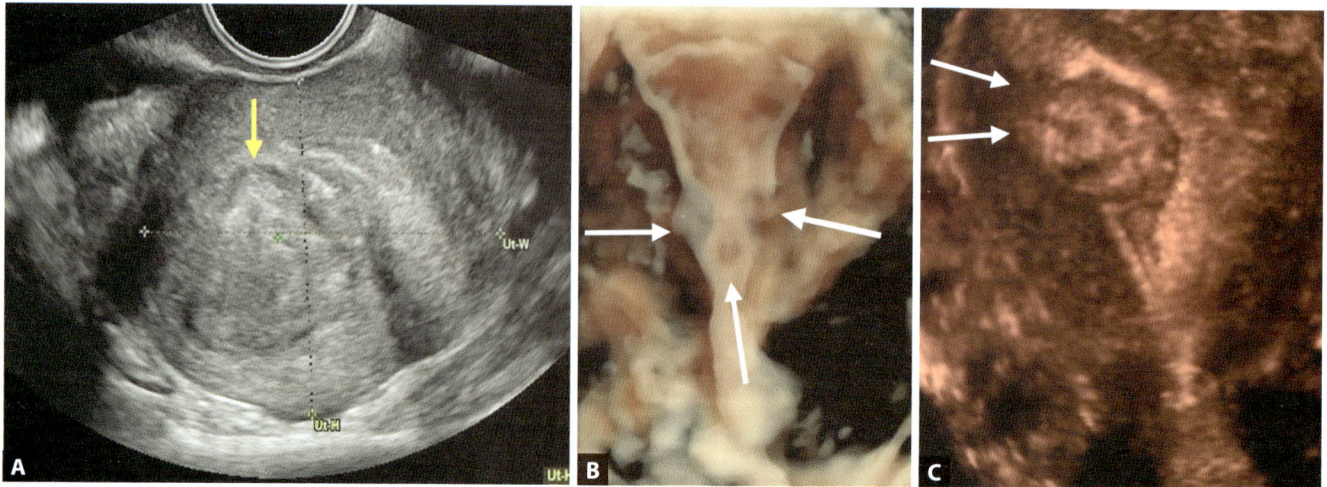

Figs. 6A to C: (A) B-mode image of endometrial fibroid (yellow arrow); (B) Multiple subendometrial fibroids, as shown by arrows on 3D ultrasound; (C) Subendometrial fibroid as shown by arrows on 3D US rendered image.

TABLE 1: Ultrasound features to differentiate endometrial polyps from type 0 fibroids.

Ultrasound features	Polyp	Endometrial fibroid
Echogenicity	Echogenic	Hypoechoic
Better seen in	Proliferative phase	Secretory phase
Vascularity	Single feeder	Peripheral
Junctional zone	Intact	Infolded
Angle between lesion and endometrium	Acute	Obtuse

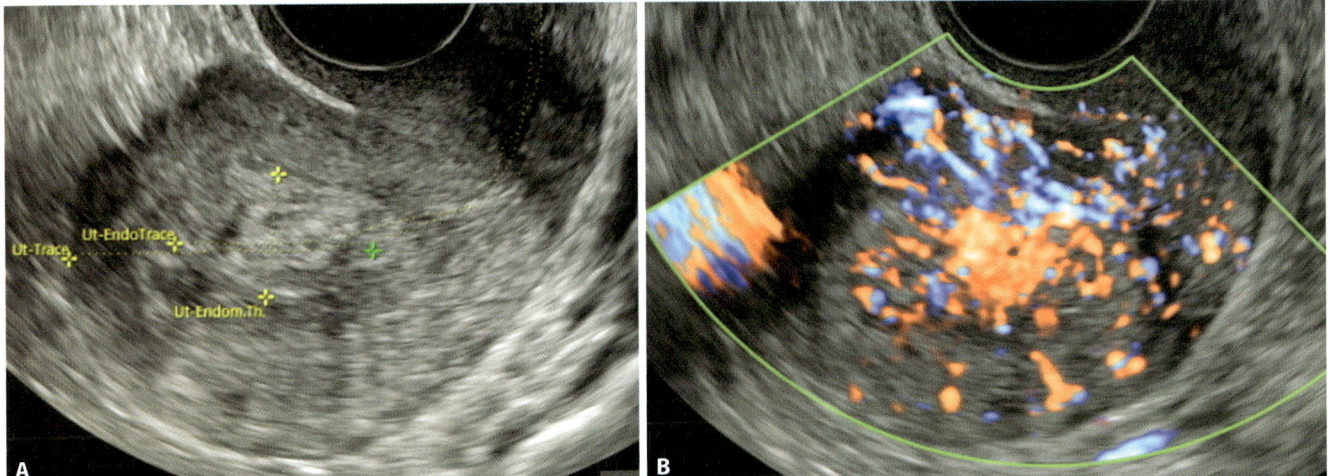

Figs. 7A and B: (A) 2D ultrasound image of thickened heterogeneous ultrasound with obliterated junctional zone; (B) On power Doppler, this lesion shows heterogeneously distributed vascularity—both suggestive of endometrial malignancy.

subendometrial or endometrial polyps. Depending on the penetration, these are divided into types 0, 1, and 2—completely inside the endometrium, more than 50% in the endometrium, and less than 50% in the endometrium, respectively. Being fibroids, these are hypoechoic to myometrium, round or oval, well defined with peripheral vascularity on Doppler. However, type 0 fibroids need to be differentiated from polyps **(Table 1)**.

- *Fibroid polyps:* These are broad-based solid heterogeneously echogenic lesion, with myometrial interface towards polyp wall and with single feeder arising from radial arteries.
- *Endometrial malignancy* **(Figs. 7A and B)**: Thickened heterogeneous endometrium in US with obliterated or inaccessible junctional zone and heterogeneously distributed hypervascularity are typical US features of endometrial malignancy. Vessels show asymmetrical caliber and abundant dichotomous branching with low-resistance flow. 3D power Doppler is an efficient modality for the study of this typically malignant vascular pattern.

■ SUMMARY

Transvaginal US is the modality of choice for assessment of the endometrium and diagnosis of endometrial pathologies. Doppler is an essential addition for the differential diagnosis of these pathologies because of the specific vascular patterns of different endometrial pathologies. Sonohysterography and 3D US play an important role in the demonstration of endometrial lesions. 3D power Doppler especially is of importance for diagnosis, assessing the extent, and follow-up of malignant lesions.

Chapter 13

Miscellaneous Uterine Lesions

Miscellaneous uterine lesions may be related to:
- Uterine scars and isthmocele
- Intrauterine device (IUD)

UTERINE SCARS AND ISTHMOCELES

Cesarean section (CS) scar is common on the uterine body and is quite similar in majority of the patients **(Fig. 1)**. Lately, incidence of cesarean deliveries has increased and with that its complications have also become more evident. Apart from the cesarean scar pregnancy and the abnormally adherent placenta, weak cesarean scar is also a major problem in patients still desiring future pregnancy. Weakened scar hosts a fluid collection and is named as "isthmocele" **(Fig. 2)**.

An isthmocele, or uterine niche, **(Fig. 3)** is any indentation representing myometrial discontinuity or a triangular anechoic defect in the anterior uterine wall, with the base communicating to the uterine cavity, at the site of a previous CS scar.

It is believed that isthmocele is more common when CS is done on the uterus that has undergone curettage

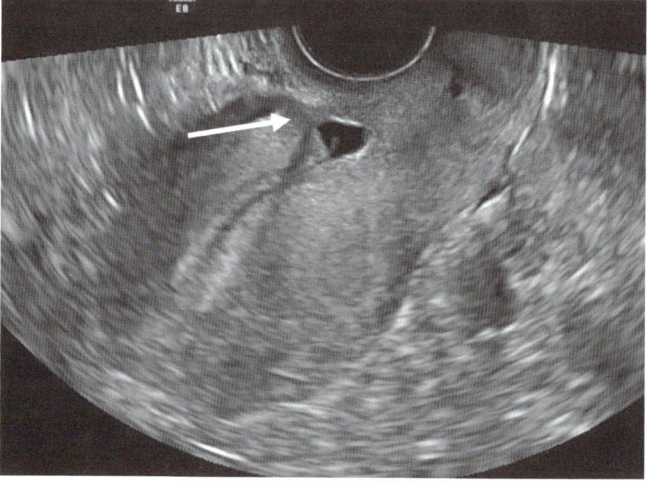

Fig. 2: B-mode ultrasound image of the midsagittal section of the uterus showing isthmocele (white arrow).

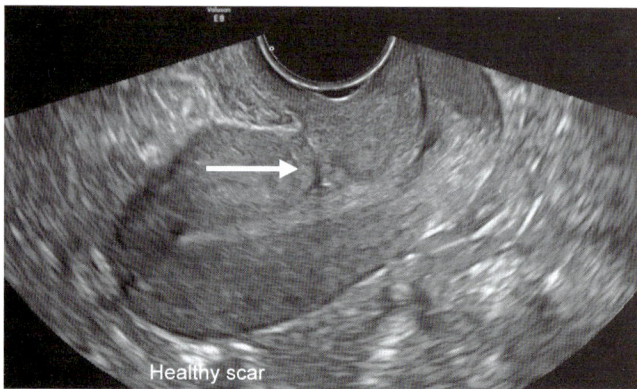

Fig. 1: B-mode ultrasound image of the midsagittal section of the uterus showing a healthy scar (white arrow).

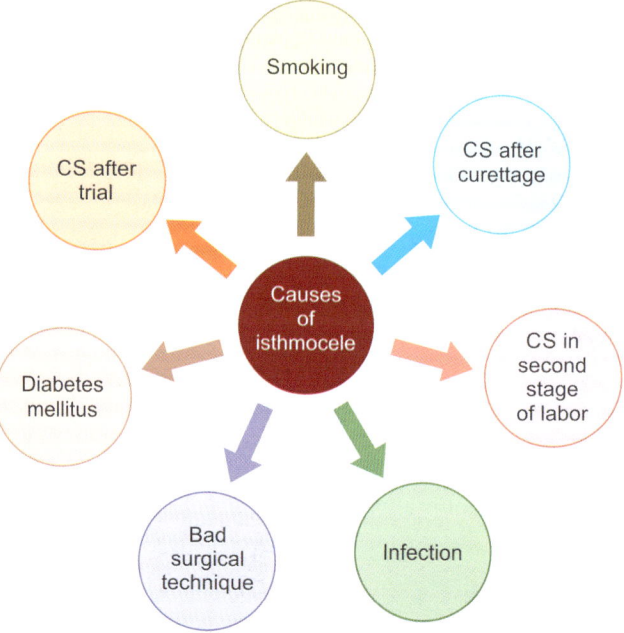

Fig. 3: Causes of isthmocele. (CS: cesarean section)

earlier, when CS is done late in the second stage of labor, after a trial, without removing the previous scar; surgical closure is done in single layer, without closing the peritoneum leading to adhesions between incision and anterior abdominal wall. Sometimes, it is caused when incision is placed on the cervix when dilatation is >5 cm and is too low and may include cervical mucous glands in scar. Even too-tight suturing can lead to necrosis and tearing off of tissues and cause a weak scar. Apart from the causes related to technique, infection, smoking, healing by second intention, and diabetes mellitus are also causative of a weak scar.

This may lead to abnormal uterine blood loss, dysmenorrhea, chronic pelvic pain, dyspareunia, subfertility, placenta accreta or previa, scar dehiscence and uterine rupture, scar ectopic pregnancy, etc.

When a weak scar **(Figs. 4A and B)** or an isthmocele is seen, it should be reported under following heads **(Fig. 5)**:
- Shape
- Scar thickness (thickening)
- Continuity of myometrium
- Border scar out
- Echoing the structure of the lower uterine segment
- Scar volume
- The residual myometrial thickness (RMT) and the shape of the scar are the most important criteria that decide the prognosis of future pregnancy in case of isthmocele.

Signs that indicate that the myometrium is adequate for vaginal delivery:
- *V shape* of the lower uterine segment

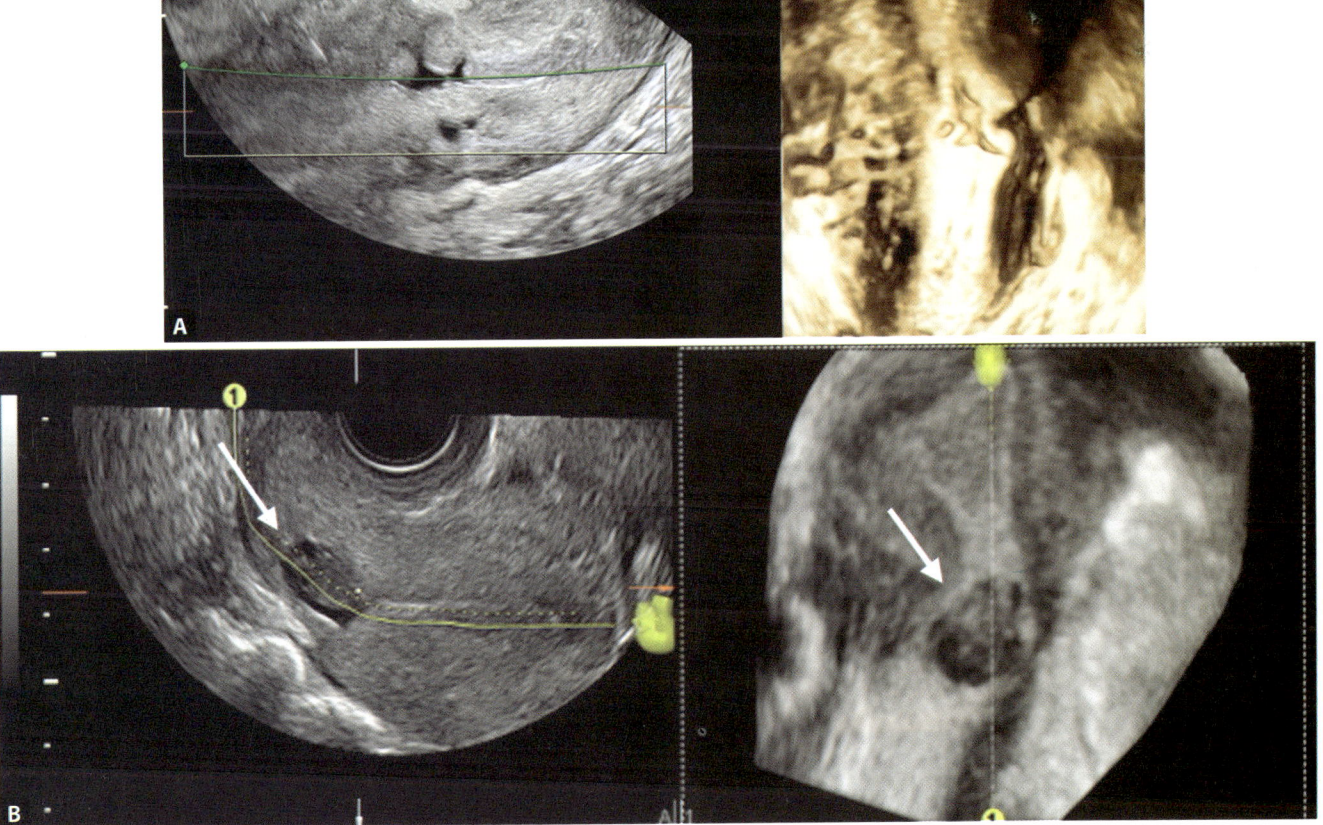

Figs. 4A and B: (A) B-mode and 3D ultrasound rendered image of weak uterine scar; (B) B-mode and 3D ultrasound rendered image of a weak uterine scar communicating with the peritoneal cavity (white arrow).

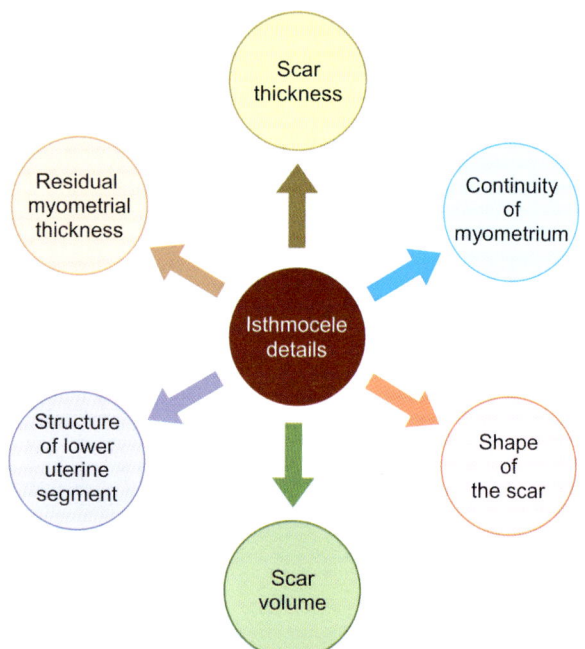

Fig. 5: Measurements to be taken for reporting of isthmocele.

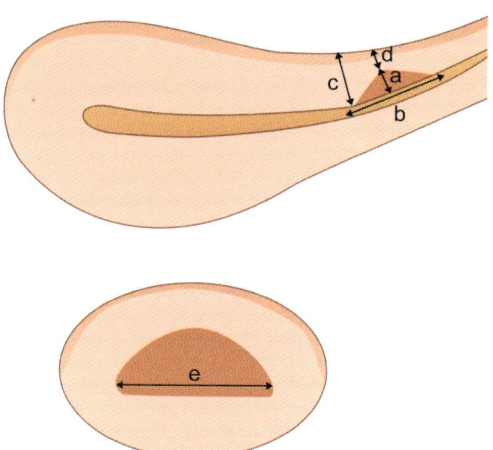

Fig. 6: Measurements taken for isthmocele. a—height of the defect (isthmocele), b—length of the defect, c—myometrial thickness just above the isthmocele, d—residual myometrial thickness at the level of isthmocele, e—width of isthmocele in transverse section.

- Minimum *thickness of 3–4 mm*
- *Continuous contour* of the lower uterine segment
- *Homogeneous echo structure*
- Or, structures with small areas of increased echogenicity

Signs that indicate that vaginal delivery may lead to uterine rupture:
- *Balloon-like shape* of the lower uterine segment
- Thickness *<3 mm*
- *Discontinuity of uterine structures*
- Predominance of areas of *increased echogenicity* in the scar[1]

As for the pregnancy continuation, different studies indicate a minimum myometrial thickness of 3–3.5 cm.[2,3]

Measurement of niche depth:
- Length
- Residual myometrial thickness
- Base width (BW)
- RMT/depth ratio in sagittal section (ratio <1 denotes scar weakness with more liability for dehiscence)
- RMT in coronal plane/niche width in coronal plane ratio (ratio <1 denotes scar weakness with more liability for dehiscence)[4]

Measurement of niche/RMT in pregnancy **(Fig. 6)**:
- For the second and third trimester, measure the thickness at the thinnest part of the myometrium.
- Measure from the urine–bladder interface to the inner margin of myometrium.
- Do not include placenta.
- <4.5 cm in second and <3.5 cm in third trimester may be considered unsafe.

But still, the knowledge of this pathology is in its infancy, and the exact relationship of causes and consequences to the size and shape of isthmocele still needs further studies.

■ INTRAUTERINE DEVICES

Intrauterine devices have been long used for contraception. The one most commonly used for mechanical contraception is Copper-T, but there used to be loops also and the one commonly used for hormonal contraception is "Mirena". All the devices used have a typical shape and these are easily visible on ultrasound and identifiable by their shape **(Figs. 7A and B)**. Though generally inert, these devices may get displaced and may lead to problems like unwanted pregnancies, abnormal uterine bleeding, and occasionally pain. These may also break sometimes and the broken pieces may get lost in the body. At times these maybe forgotten after placement and maybe discovered incidentally on ultrasound of the pelvis. Ultrasound plays a major role in confirming the placement and position of intrauterine contraceptive devices (IUCDs). Displacement of IUCD is considered when there is a distance of <3 mm between the IUD and the uterine fundus, which was initially thought to be associated with a high risk of expulsion **(Figs. 8A and B)**.

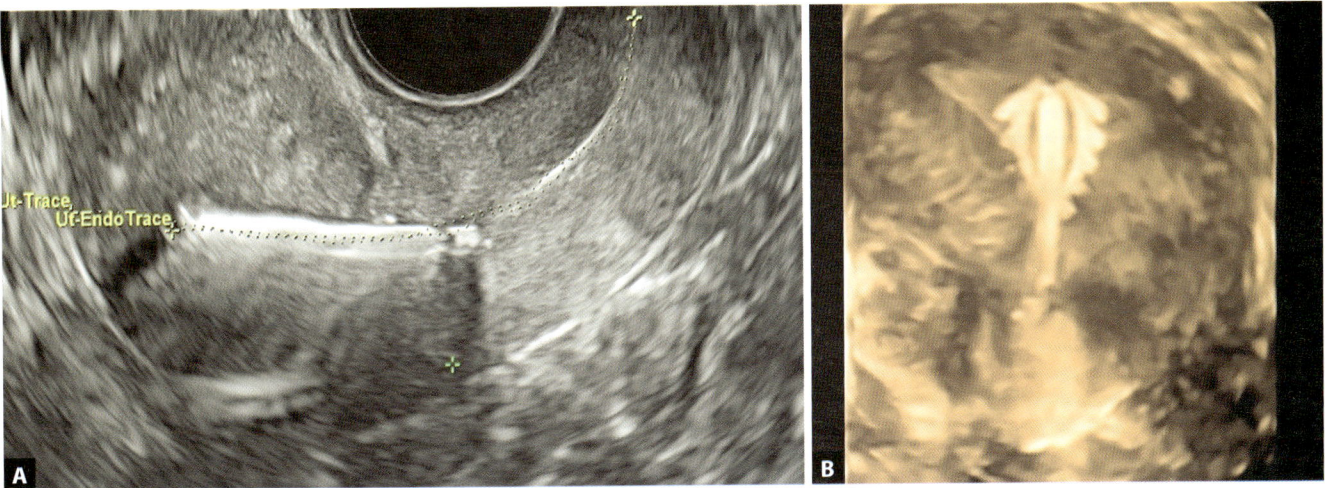

Figs. 7A and B: (A) B-mode ultrasound; (B) 3D ultrasound image of intrauterine contraceptive device (IUCD) in situ.

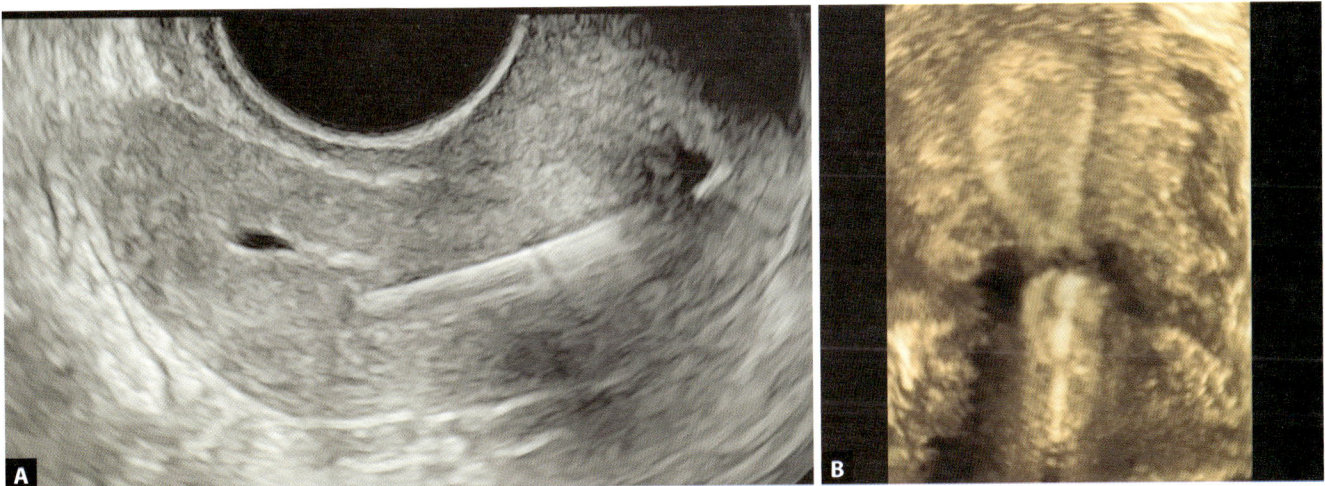

Figs. 8A and B: (A) B-mode; (B) 3D ultrasound image of displaced IUCD.

Penetration into myometrium by the arm or stem of the IUD without extension through the serosa is called embedment. When involving the stem, this may be obvious on standard 2D transvaginal ultrasound (TVUS), but in cases of more subtle arm embedment, 3D coronal images allow for better detection.

When it penetrates through the serosa, it is perforated IUCD, either partially or completely with migration into the intraperitoneal cavity. Embedment and perforation may occur at the time of insertion.

IUDs may, rarely, be broken during expulsion or removal, including embedded retrieval strings. Few data are available on the long-term effects of retained strings or pieces of devices and no clear management guidelines have been established.

Incrustation, the formation of calcium carbonate deposits on or near the IUD, is a well-described phenomenon that can be demonstrated as uneven echoes surrounding the normal IUD echoes.

SUMMARY

Isthmocele is a weak uterine scar, most commonly due to CS, and may usually result from poor surgical technique, cesarean done at the wrong time, or healing of the scar by second intention. It may lead to a risk of uterine rupture in subsequent pregnancy along with less serious presentations like bleeding, dyspareunia, dysmenorrhea, chronic pelvic pain, etc. Proper assessment of these scars' weakness by ultrasound can decide on the line of treatment.

The IUCDs can be seen on ultrasound clearly and so their complications like embedment, perforation, fragmentation, and calcification can all be diagnosed by ultrasound.

REFERENCES

1. Lebedev VA, Strizhakov AN, Zhelnezov BI. [Echographic and morphological parallels in the evaluation of the condition of the uterine scar.] Akush Ginekol (Mosk). 1991; 8:44-9.
2. Flamm BL, Lim OW, Jones C, Fallon D, Newman LA, Mantis JK. Vaginal birth after cesarean section: Results of a multicenter study. Am J Obstet Gynecol. 1998;158(5): 1079-84.
3. Wang CB, Chiu WWC, Lee CY, Sun YL, Lin YH, Tseng CJ. Cesarean scar defect: correlation between Cesarean section number, defect size, clinical symptoms and uterine position. Ultrasound Obstet Gynecol. 2009; 34(1):85-9.
4. Alafy M, Osman OM, Salama S, Lasheen Y, Soliman M, Fikry M, et al. Int J Womens Health. 2020;12:965-74.

Benign Cervical Pathologies

INTRODUCTION

The cervix is an organ easily assessable by direct visualization, examination by per speculum, and per vaginal examination, but as is well known, these chiefly assess only the external os and the distal part of the cervix. Especially, the supravaginal part of the cervix and the internal os cannot be assessed by per vaginal or per speculum examination. Moreover, lesions in the cervical canal can also not be diagnosed by this method.

Assessment of the cervix is indicated for gynecological indications like cervical polyps, cervical fibroids, cervical malignancies, and cervical ectopic pregnancy. In obstetric cases, of course, the major concern is the cervical competence and the length to assess the risk of premature labor. Of course, the cervical assessment is also important to assess the progress of the labor. But in this chapter, we shall limit our discussion to the gynecological and prelabor indications of cervical assessment.

TIPS TO ASSESS THE CERVIX

It is important to actively evaluate the ultrasound image at all times since the probe is on the introitus and slides in the vaginal canal. As it touches the cervix, gently slide the probe into anterior fornix if the uterus is anteverted–anteflexed and in the posterior fornix if it is retroverted–retroflexed. When the entire cervix is located, manipulate the probe to bring it at the center and adjust the depth so that the cervix fills at least half, preferably two-third of the image **(Figs. 1A and B)**. Then take off the pressure a bit so that the pressure on the cervical canal is released and the cervical canal opens up. Span from right to left. Rotate the probe 90° anticlockwise and span it anteroposteriorly to evaluate the cervix from internal os to external os. Finally, check the cervix for mobility. In cases, where there are doubts about cervical morphology, gel vaginosonography may be helpful.

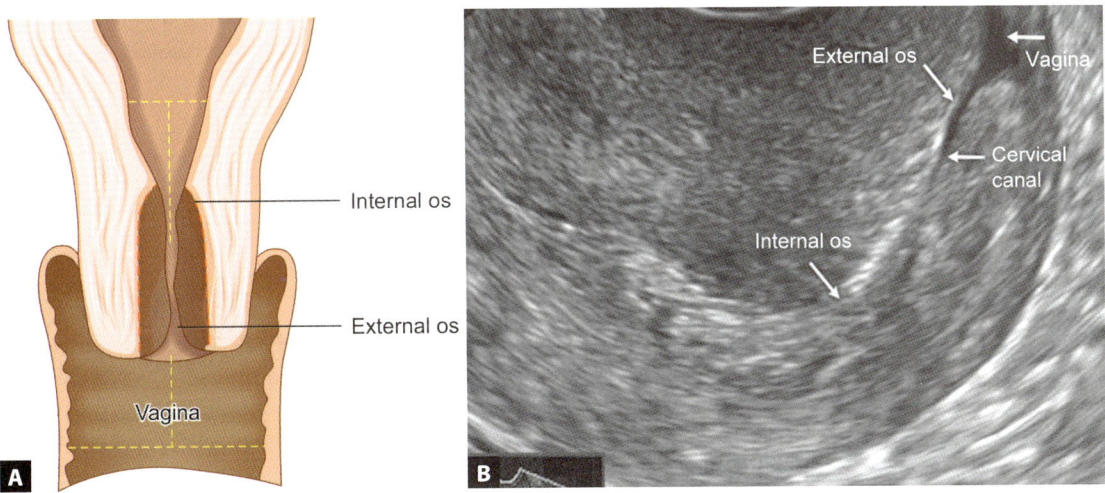

Figs. 1A and B: (A) Diagrammatic representation; (B) B-mode ultrasound image showing the anatomy of cervix.

CERVICAL POLYPS

The polyps appear as solid echogenic lesions in the cervical canal and are usually associated with fluid in the cervical canal, and so are easy to identify **(Figs. 2A to F)**. When there is no fluid in the cervical canal, these are difficult to identify but are suspected when the cervical canal

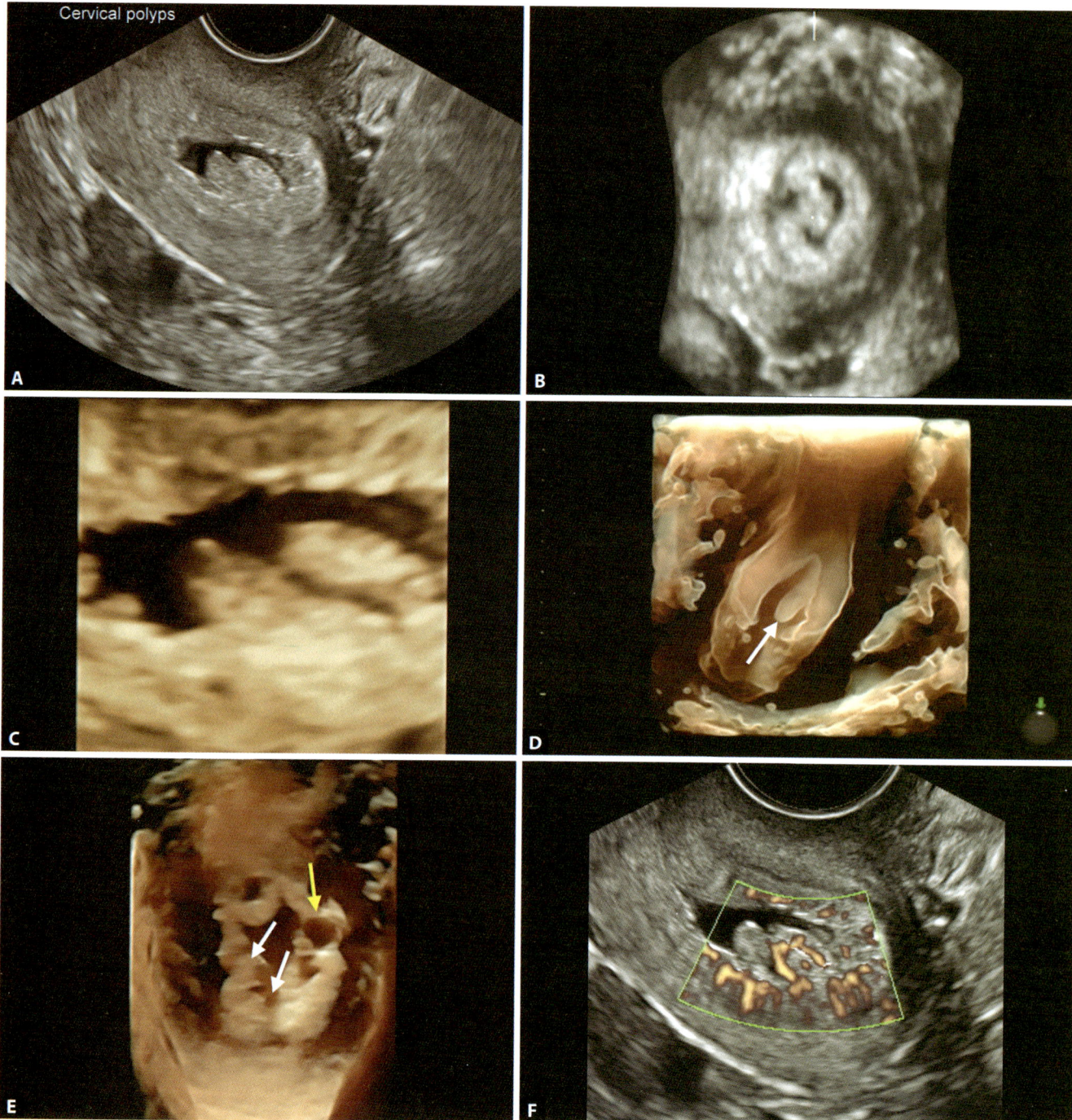

Figs. 2A to F: B-mode ultrasound image of (A) longitudinal and (B) transverse section of the cervix. Both images show fluid in a cervical canal with two solid projections in the lumen polyps; (C) 3D rendered image of the same; (D) 3D ultrasound rendered image of the cervix in coronal section shows polyp projecting in the cervical canal (white arrow); (E) 3D rendered coronal image of the cervix shows fluid in the cervical canal with multiple small papillary projections, suggestive of multiple small cervical polyps (white arrows), yellow arrow indicates Nabothian cyst; (F) Power Doppler showing feeder vessel in an individual polyp.

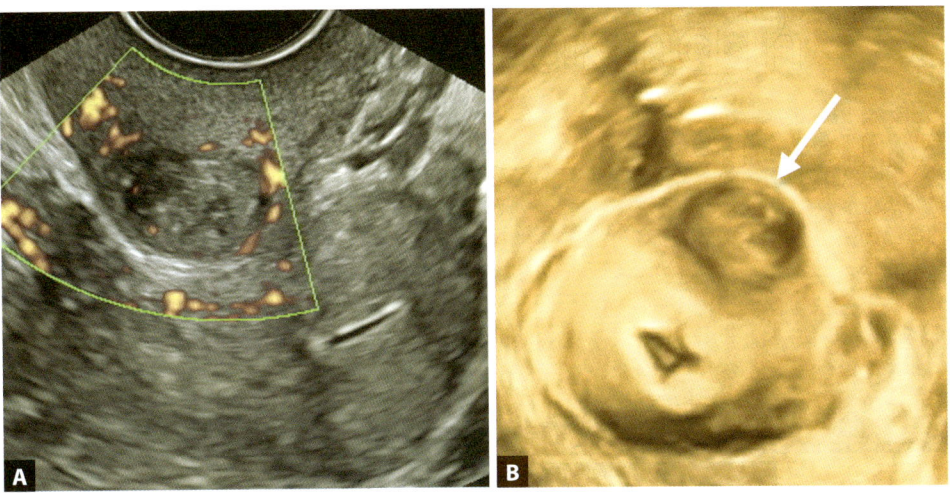

Figs. 3A and B: (A) B-mode with power Doppler image of cervical fibroid; (B) 3D ultrasound image of cervical fibroid (white arrow).

Shows irregularity. On color or power Doppler, these polyps typically show single-feeding vessel pattern like endometrial polyps **(Figs. 2A and B)**. Cervical polyps, when small, are not of much clinical significance, but when large, may lead to obstruction for the passage of intrauterine insemination cannula or embryo-transfer cannula.

■ CERVICAL FIBROIDS

Cervical fibroids are not very common. These fibroids are also hypoechoic round or oval well-defined lesions like uterine fibroids and also show peripheral rim-like vascularity **(Figs. 3A and B)**. When more than one-half of the fibroid extent is below the internal os, this fibroid can be called cervical fibroid. Though these are usually classified as type eight of International Federation of Gynecology and Obstetrics (FIGO)/PALM–COEIN (*p*olyp, *a*denomyosis, *l*eiomyoma, *m*alignancy and hyperplasia, *c*oagulopathy, *o*vulatory dysfunction, *e*ndometrial, *i*atrogenic, and *n*ot yet classified) Classification, their penetration needs to be mentioned in relation to cervical mucosa or serosa.

■ NABOTHIAN CYSTS

The Nabothian cysts are very common in cervix **(Fig. 4)**. These are well-defined roundish or oval cystic lesions. These are dilatation of cervical glands due to the collection of secretions of cervical glands. Generally, Nabothian cysts are not of much significance, but when the contents are echogenic, there may be an indication of severe infection and these patients may present with foul-smelling vaginal

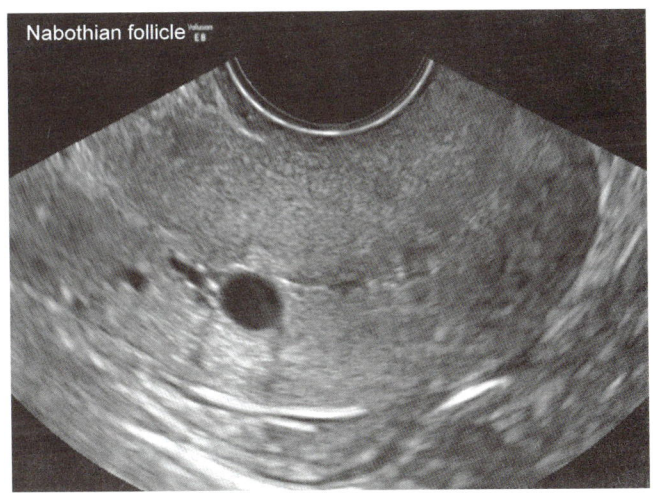

Fig. 4: Anechoic cystic lesion in the cervix, adjacent to cervical canal—Nabothian cyst.

discharge. Nabothian cysts are not a cause of infertility and unless multiple and large, may not even lead to mechanical obstruction.

■ SUMMARY

Cervix is easily approachable clinically but still lesions in the cervical canal and deep in the cervical wall are difficult to diagnose on clinical assessment only and are a cause of concern for intermittent bleeding, vaginal discharge, etc. Ultrasound is a tool of choice for confirmatory diagnosis. Especially when probe manipulation allows separation of the walls of the cervix, or by gel vaginosonography, diagnosis of lesions within the cervical canal become clearly visible. Doppler can be of additional help.

Cervical Length Assessment and Elasticity

Cervical assessment is important for gynecological and obstetric indications **(Table 1)**.

METHODS OF CERVICAL ASSESSMENT FOR OBSTETRIC CASES

Though the cervix is an organ easy to access clinically, supravaginal part of the cervix cannot be assessed clinically. Ultrasound gives information about cervical length and also about cervical dilatation. This can be done by transabdominal, transperineal, translabial, or transvaginal route. Translabial or transperineal ultrasound is not always able to provide adequate information on the cervix because of maternal obesity or because of acoustic shadowing from the rectum or symphysis pubis. This acoustic shadowing even when does not obliterate the visualization completely, may obscure the cervical canal partially and result in false shortening of cervical length.[1]

For transabdominal assessment of the cervix, the bladder needs to be full; this stretches the cervix resulting in apparent lengthening of the cervix.[2] Transvaginal ultrasound is the modality of choice for assessment of the cervix **(Flowcharts 1 and Fig. 1)**. Cervical length is measured as the distance from internal os to external os. Transvaginal ultrasonography can help identify the presence of other ultrasound risk markers for preterm

TABLE 1: Gynecological and obstetric indications from assessment of the cervix.

Gynecological indications	Obstetric indications
Cervical polyp	Cervical incompetence
Cervical fibroid	Assessing risk of premature labor and planning cerclage
Cervical malignancy	Predict successful labor
Cervical ectopic pregnancy	

Flowchart 1: Assessment of cervical length on ultrasound.

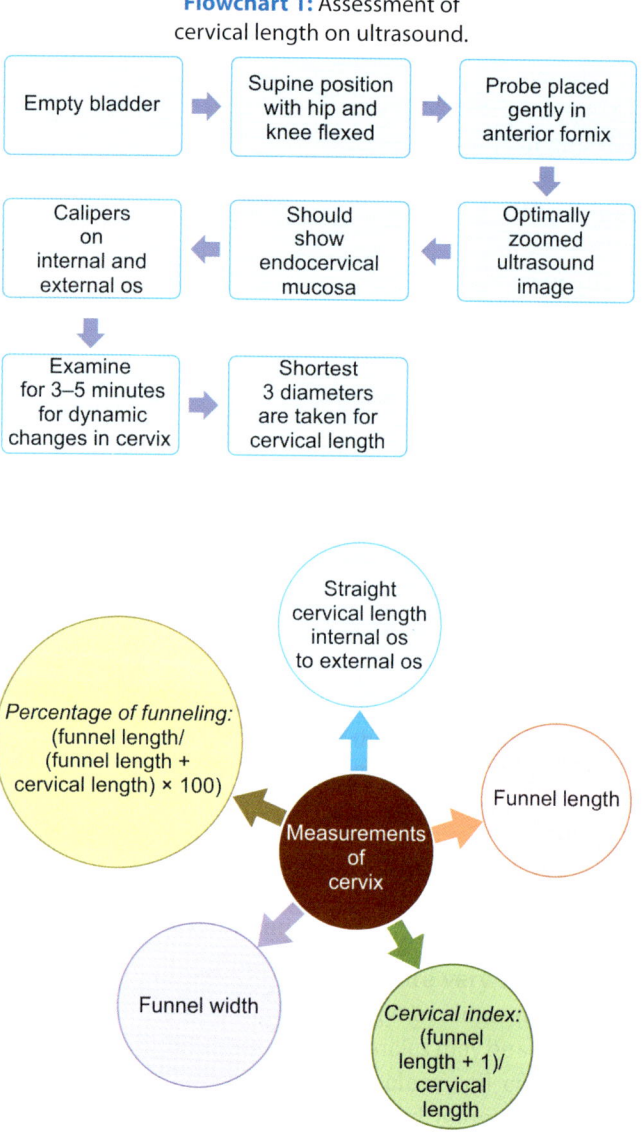

Fig. 1: Different measurements to be taken during cervical assessment.

delivery, such as the presence of intra-amniotic debris (a possible sign of intrauterine microbial colonization) and choriodecidual separation.[3]

A dynamic assessment of the cervical length with and without fundal pressure is a more reliable method for assessment of cervical incompetence in women at high risk, at 15–24 weeks.[4] MacDonald et al. reported that opening of the internal os at rest or in response to transfundal pressure as the earliest ultrasound feature of cervical incompetence.[4,5]

Technique

An algorithm for assessment of cervical length on ultrasound is given in **Flowchart 1**.

The caliper for internal os is placed at the apex of V-shaped notch and for external os, it is placed at the apex of triangular echodensity of external os.[6]

The criteria that are mandatory for cervical length assessment are as follows:
- Internal os should be clearly visible as flat dimple or as hypoechoic triangle.
- Whole length of cervical canal should be clearly visible.
- External os should appear symmetrical.
- External surface of the cervix should be clearly identified.
- Distance from posterior lip of cervical canal should be identical to distance from anterior lip. When this technique for cervical length assessment is followed, the interobserver error is 5–10%.

Difficulties for Cervical Assessment

The difficulties include the following:
- Undeveloped lower uterine segment and difficult-to-identify internal os
- Focal myometrial contraction
- Rapid and spontaneous cervical change
- Endocervical polyps
- Incorrect interpretation for dilatation of internal os due to vaginal probe orientation
- Artificial lengthening of the cervical canal due to distortion of cervix by the transducer[7]

CERVICAL INSUFFICIENCY

If the cervix is to be measured in the first trimester, measure the linear distance between the two ends of glandular area of cervix and then measure the shortest distance between the glandular area and the gestational sac (isthmic length).[8]

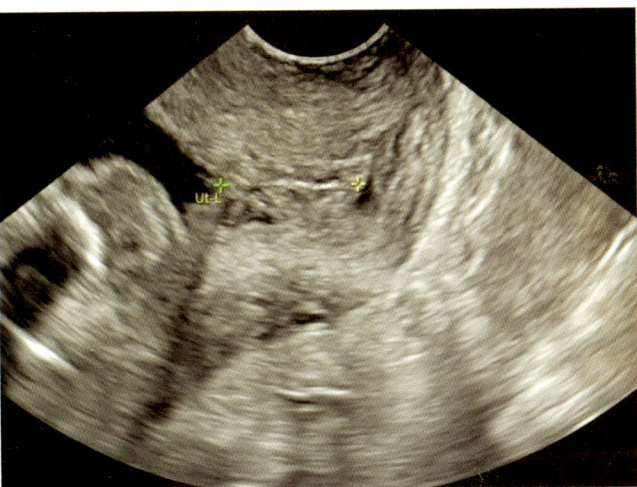

Fig. 2: Cervical length measurement in second trimester.

Serial measurements of cervix in first and second trimesters and the rate of decrease in cervical length may be useful to assess the risk of preterm delivery **(Fig. 2)**.

Transvaginal cervical assessment for prediction of preterm birth was first documented by Anderson et al. This study had shown that a cervical length of <39 mm before 30 weeks of pregnancy was a significant risk factor for early delivery.[9]

By other workers, it is defined on transvaginal sonography (TVS) as cervical length <25 mm and/or advanced cervical changes on physical examination before 24 weeks of gestation in women with either one or more prior pregnancy losses or preterm births at 14–36 weeks.

In women with a history of spontaneous preterm birth, a systematic review of controlled studies showed that measurement of cervical length in the second trimester, especially before 24 weeks, predicted the risk of recurrent preterm birth[10] and has sensitivity of 65.4%, specificity of 75.5%, positive predictive value (PPV) of 33.0%, and negative predictive value (NPV) of 92.0%.

Whereas another study showed a sensitivity of 56%, PPV of 90%, specificity of 96%, and NPV of 79% for preterm delivery with cervical length of ≤20 mm. Cervical measurement before 16 weeks is not a reliable screening method for assessing the risk of preterm delivery because internal os is not identifiable.[11]

The shorter the cervical length, the higher the positive likelihood ratio for spontaneous preterm birth at <35 weeks.[12]

But this is not an assurance that pregnancy problems of abortions or preterm labor will not occur if cervical length is normal. However, if the cervix is short, it definitely depicts early abortion or labor.

Frequency of Examination

In women with prior preterm birth at 28–36 weeks, it is recommended to initiate screening at 16 weeks. Ultrasound examination is generally repeated every 2 weeks until 24 weeks as long as the cervical length is ≥30 mm and increased to weekly if the cervical length is 25–29 mm, with the expectation that preterm cervical changes will precede overt preterm labor or membrane rupture symptoms by 3–6 weeks.[12]

Cervical ultrasonography appears to be more efficient as a short-term than as a long-term predictor, so serial examinations in a time interval of 10–14 days for women with short cervical length should be recommended.[13]

Multiple regression analysis has confirmed that cervical length was a significant predictor of preterm birth before 35 weeks and that multiparous had a 43% greater risk compared with nulliparous.[14] Transvaginal scan for cervical measurement at 22–24 weeks, has shown TVS to be superior to Bishop score and fetal fibronectin in cervicovaginal secretion. But at 31–32 weeks, no one method is better than the other for predicting preterm delivery.[15]

For singleton pregnancy, the cutoff for the exponential rise in risk of preterm delivery is 15 mm, whereas for multiple pregnancies, it is 25 mm.[16] Although when the cervix is shorter than 15 mm at the time of cerclage at 22–24 weeks, the risk of delivery before 33 weeks cannot be substantially reduced.[17]

In women with *symptoms of preterm labor*, it is not possible by frequency or intensity of contractions to differentiate between true and false preterm labor.[18] Transvaginal ultrasound can assess the cervix and differentiate between the two and can also predict preterm delivery.

Funneling must be documented. It is described as Y- or U-shape of cervix and is a good predictor of preterm delivery in second trimester, but may be normally seen after 32 weeks.[19] Although To et al. concluded that funneling did not provide a significant additional contribution to cervical length in prediction of delivery before 33 weeks.[20]

In patients with threatened preterm labor, cervical length of <30 mm had a high risk of preterm delivery and those with <20 mm of cervical length delivered preterm.[21] Presence of cervical funneling of >75% or a cervical shortening of <10 mm was predictive of preterm premature rupture of membranes (PPROM).[22] In patients with PPROM, cervical length of <20 mm and/or funneling (Fig. 3) was associated with short-time interval from admission to delivery.[23] Short cervix and/or funneling can be used as a guide to decide on tocolytic therapy. In one of the largest studies of 3,694 singleton pregnancies, cervical assessment was done. When cervical length was <29 mm between 18 and 22 weeks, the relative risk for delivery before 35 weeks was 8 as compared to 28 when internal os was dilated to 5 mm.[24]

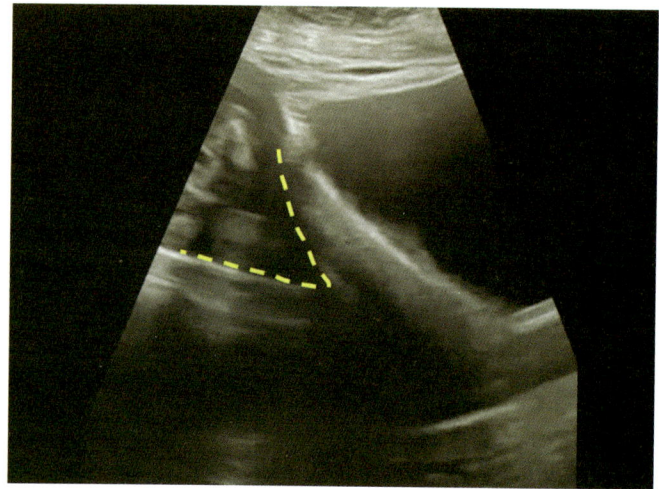

Fig. 3: Dashed lines showing cervical funneling.

Impact on Management

Elective cervical cerclage has a significant effect in preventing spontaneous preterm birth before 34 weeks of gestation.[24] Placement of cervical cerclage before 27 weeks of gestation in women who have a cervix shorter than 25 mm may reduce the incidence of preterm delivery before 34 weeks of gestation among high-risk patients.[17] In a nonhigh-risk population, a single TVS cervical length measurement should be done at 18–24 weeks in women with risk factors for cervical insufficiency and no prior delivery, and treat those with a short cervix (≤20 mm) with vaginal progesterone supplementation.

Because of poor values and sensitivities and a lack of proven effective interventions, routine transvaginal cervical length assessment is not recommended in women at low risk.

High-risk population for preterm delivery includes women with:

- History of preterm delivery

- Rupture of membranes
  - Repeated mid-trimester pregnancy losses
  - Cervical surgery
  - Congenital uterine abnormalities
  - Diethylstilbestrol exposure

To summarize, the assessment of the cervix in pregnant women for the risk of preterm labor include measuring the cervical length, funneling of internal os, and shortening of the cervix on dynamic examination.

REFERENCES

1. Carr DB, Smith K, Parsons L, Chansky K, Shields LE. Ultrasonography for cervical length measurement: Agreement between transvaginal and translabial techniques. Obstet Gynecol. 2000;96(4):554-8.
2. To MS, Skemtou C, Cicero S, Nicolaides KH. Cervical assessment at the routine 23 weeks scan: Problems with transabdominal sonography. Ultrasound Obstet Gynecol. 2000;15(4):292-6.
3. Kusanovic JP, Espinoza J, Romero R, Gonçalves LF, Nien JK, Soto E, et al. Clinical significance of the presence of amniotic fluid 'sludge' in asymptomatic patients at high risk for spontaneous preterm delivery. Ultrasound Obstet Gynecol. 2007;30(5):706-14.
4. MacDonald R, Smith P, Vyas S. Cervical incompetence: The use of transvaginal sonography to provide an objective diagnosis. Ultrasound Obstet Gynecol. 2001;18(3):211-6.
5. Guzman ER, Pisatowski DM, Vintzileos AM, Benito CW, Hanley ML, Ananth CV. A comparison of ultrasonographically detected cervical changes in response to transfundal pressure, coughing and standing in predicting cervical incompetence. Am J Obstet Gynecol. 1997;177(3):660-5.
6. Owen J, Iams JD; National Institute of Child Health and Human Development Maternal-Fetal Medicine Units Network. What we have learned about cervical ultrasound. Semin Perinatol. 2003;27(3):194-203.
7. Yost NP, Bloom SL, Twickler DM, Leveno KJ. Pitfalls in ultrasonographic cervical canal length measurement for predicting preterm birth. Obstet Gynecol. 1999;93(4):510-6.
8. Greco E, Lange A, Ushakov F, Calvo JR, Nicolaides KH. Prediction of spontaneous preterm delivery from endocervical length at 11–13 weeks. Prenat Diagn. 2011;31(1):84-9.
9. Anderson HF, Nugent CE, Wanty SD, Hayashi RH. Prediction of risk of preterm delivery by ultrasonographic measurement of cervical length. Am J Obstet Gynecol. 1990;163(3):859-67.
10. Crane JM, Hutchens D. Transvaginal sonographic measurement of cervical length to predict preterm birth in asymptomatic women at increased risk: A systematic review. Ultrasound Obstet Gynecol. 2008;31(5):579-87.
11. Conoscenti G, Meir YJ, D'Ottavio G, Rustico MA, Pinzano R, Fischer-Tamaro L, et al. Does cervical length at 13–15 weeks' gestation predict preterm delivery in the unselected population. Ultrasound Obstet Gynecol. 2003;21(2):128-34.
12. Iams JD, Cebrik D, Lynch C, Behendt N, Das A. The rate of cervical change and the phenotype of spontaneous preterm birth. Am J Obstet Gynecol. 2011;205(2):130.e1-6.
13. Heath VC, Southall TR, Souka AP, Elisseou A, Nicolaides KH. Cervical length at 23 weeks of gestation: Prediction of spontaneous preterm delivery. Ultrasound Obstet Gynecol. 1998;12(5):312-7.
14. Fujita MM, Brizot Mde L, Liao AW, Bernáth T, Cury L, Neto JD, et al. Reference range for cervical length in twin pregnancies. Acta Obstet Gynecol Scan. 2002;81(9):856-9.
15. Hoesli I, Tercanli S, Holzgreve W. Cervical length assessment by ultrasound as a predictor of preterm labour—is there a role for routine screening? BJOG. 2003;110(Suppl 20):61-5.
16. Berghella V, Talucci M, Desai A. Does transvaginal sonographic measurement of cervical length before 14 weeks predict preterm delivery in high risk pregnancies? Ultrasound Obstet Gynecol. 2003;21(2):140-4.
17. Crane J, Scott H, Stewart A, Chandra S, Whittle W, Hutchens D. Transvaginal ultrasonography to predict preterm birth in women with bicornuate or didelphys uterus. J Matern Fetal Neonatal Med. 2012;25(10):1960-4.
18. Iams JD, Casal D, McGregor JA, Goodwin TM, Kreaden US, Lowensohn R, et al. Fetal fibronection improves the accuracy of diagnosis of preterm labour. Am J Obstet Gynecol. 1995;173(1):141-5.
19. Barghella V, Kuhlman K, Weiner S, Texeira L, Wapner RJ. Cervical funneling: Sonographic criteria predictive of preterm delivery. Ultrasound Obstet Gynecol. 1997;10(3):161-6.
20. To MS, Skentuo C, Liao AW, Cacho A, Nicolaides KH. Cervical length and funneling at 23 weeks of gestation in the prediction of spontaneous early preterm delivery. Ultrasound Obstet Gynecol. 2001;18:200-3.
21. Murakawa H, Utumi T, Hasegawa I, Tanaka K, Fuzimori R. E. Evaluation of threatened preterm delivery by transvaginal ultrasonographic measurement of cervical length. Obstet Gynecol. 1993;82(5):829-32.
22. Obido AO, Berghella V, Reddy U, Tolosa JE, Wapner RJ. Does transvaginal ultrasound of the cervix predict preterm premature rupture of membranes in a high-risk population? Ultrasound Obstet Gynecol. 2001;18(3):223-7.
23. Carlan SJ, Richmond LB, O'brien WF. Randomized trial of endovaginal ultrasound in preterm premature rupture of membranes. Obstet Gynecol. 1997;89(3):458-61.
24. Heath VC, Southall TR, Souka AP, Novakov A, Nicolaides KH. Cervical length at 23 weeks of gestation: Relation to demographic characteristics and previous obstetric history. Ultrasound Obstet Gynecol. 1998;12(5):304-11.

Chapter 16: Common Ovarian Lesions

Flowchart 1: Classification of adnexal lesions according to ultrasound morphology.

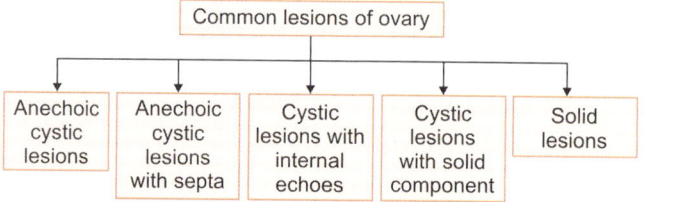

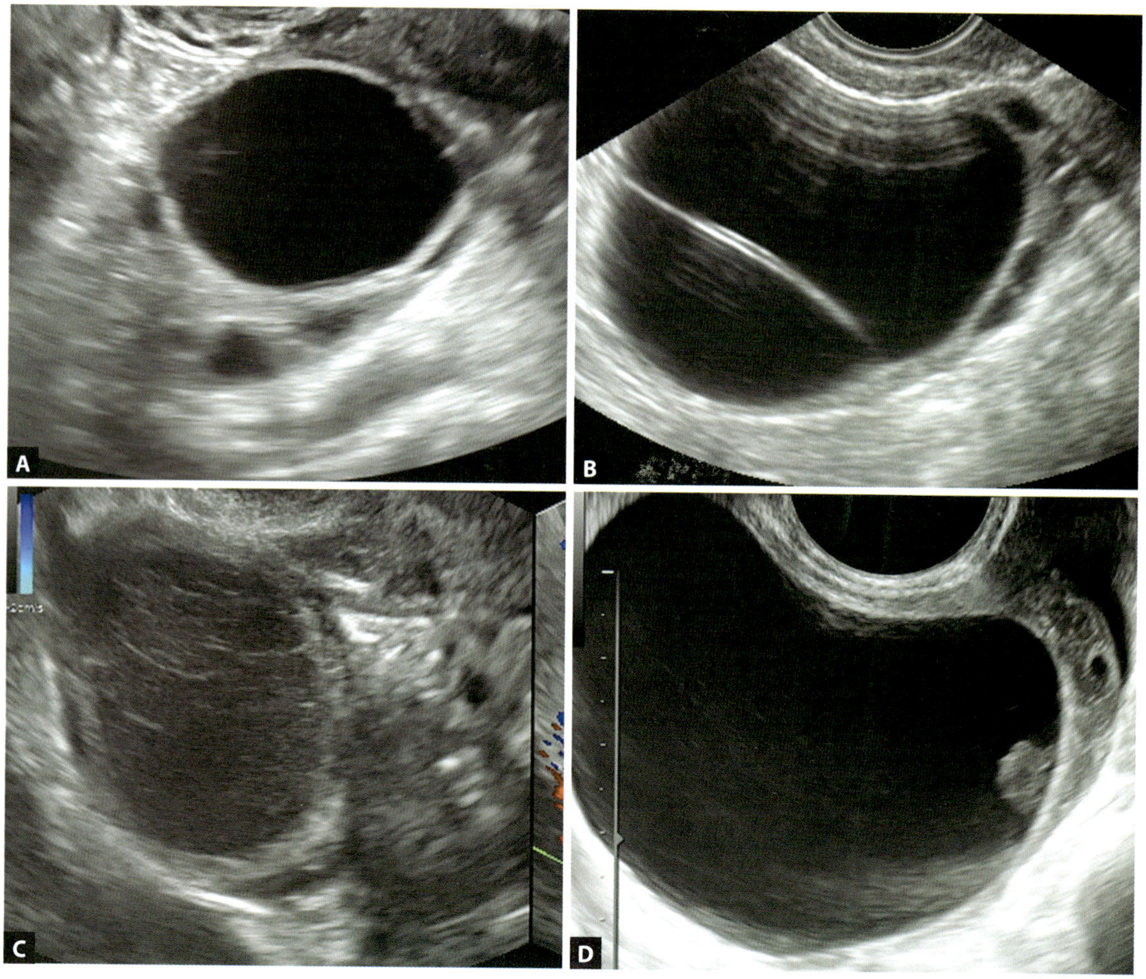

Figs. A to D

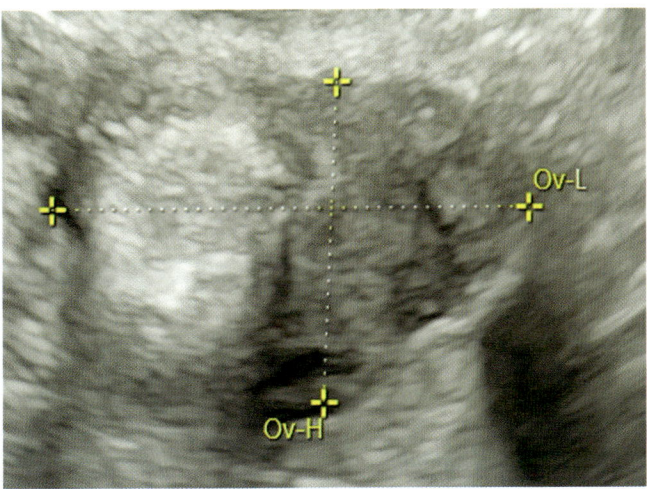

Fig. E

Figs. A to E: (A) Anechoic cystic lesion; (B) Anechoic septated cystic lesion; (C) Cystic lesion with internal echoes; (D) Cystic lesion with solid projection; (E) Solid lesion.

Flowchart 2: Differential diagnosis of intraovarian anechoic cystic lesions.

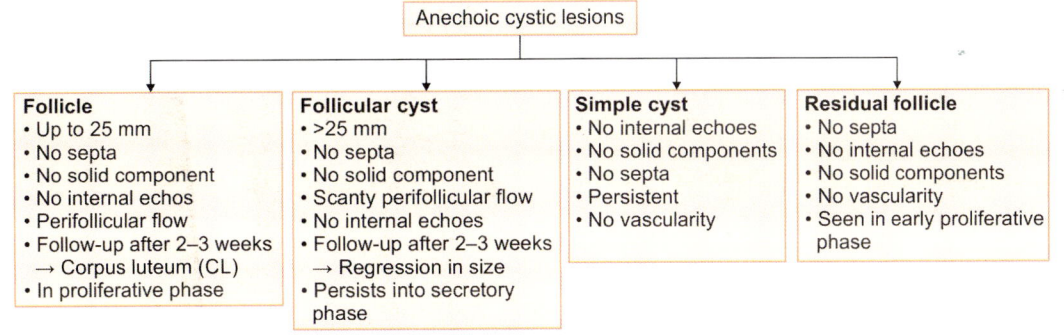

Flowchart 3: Differential diagnosis of intraovarian anechoic cystic lesions with septa.

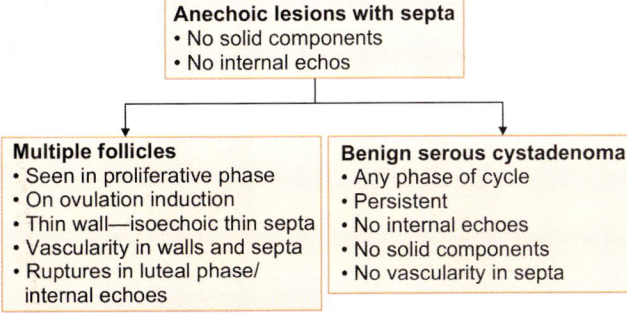

Common Ovarian Lesions

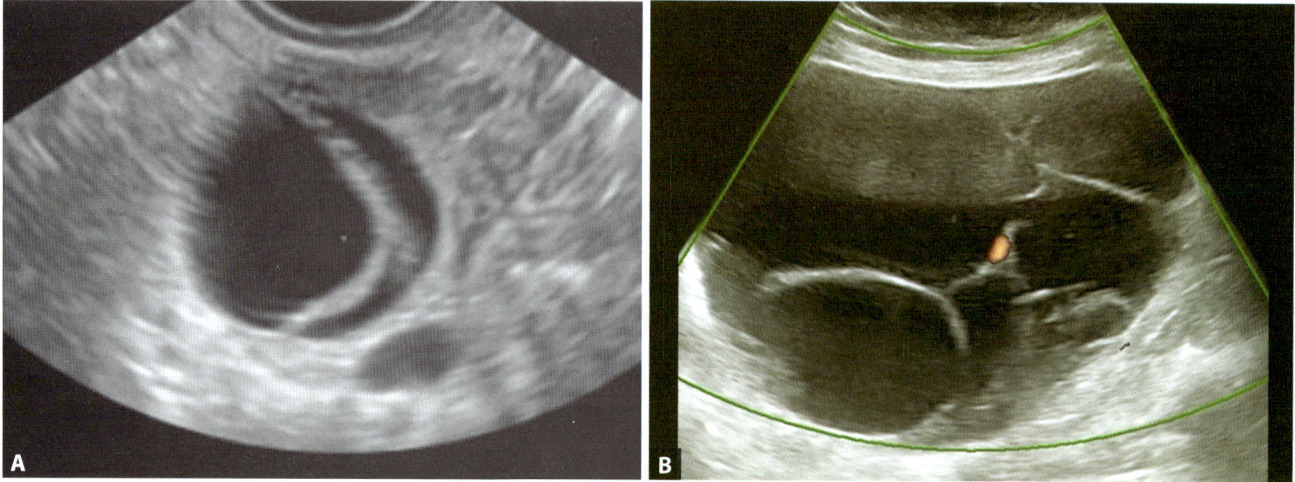

Figs. 2A and B: (A) Multiple follicles; (B) Serous cystadenoma.

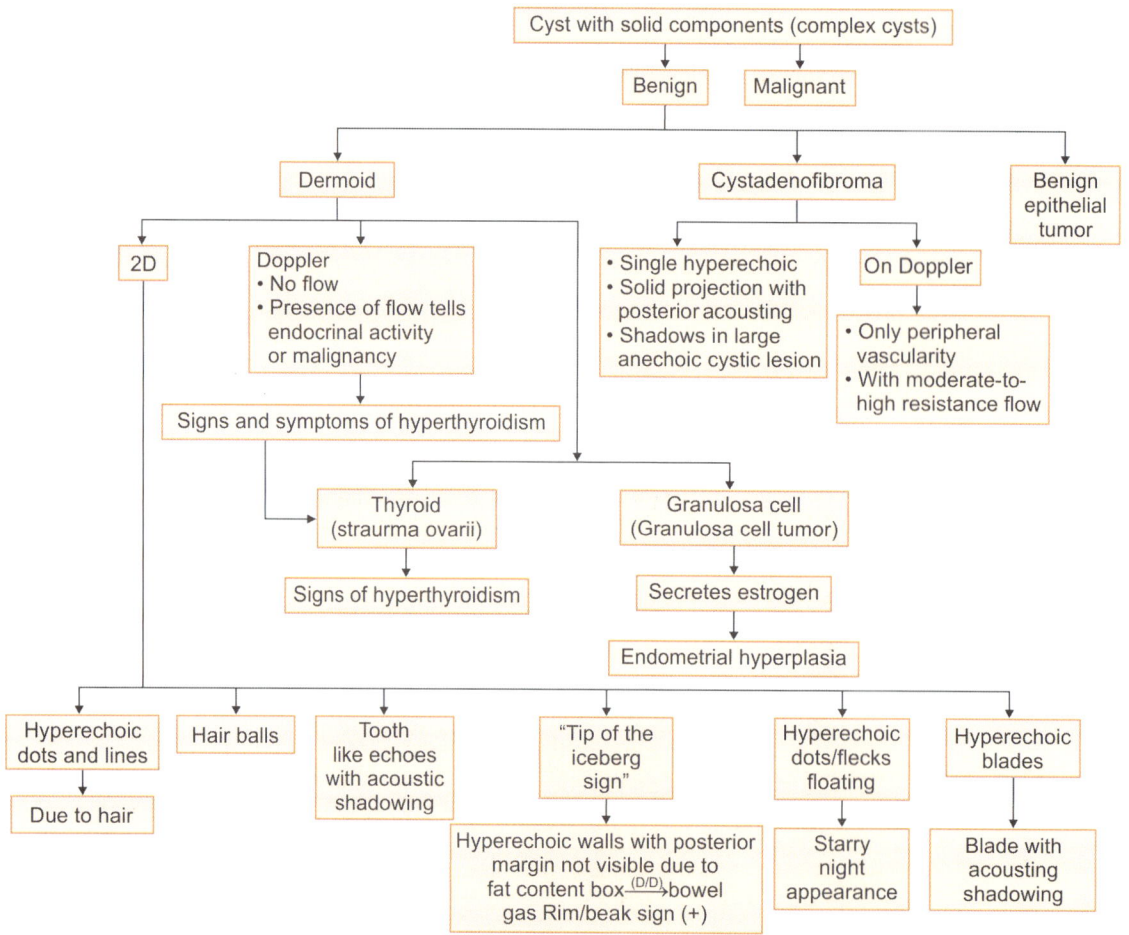

Flowchart 4: Differential diagnosis of intraovarian cystic lesions with solid components.

Common Ovarian Lesions 49

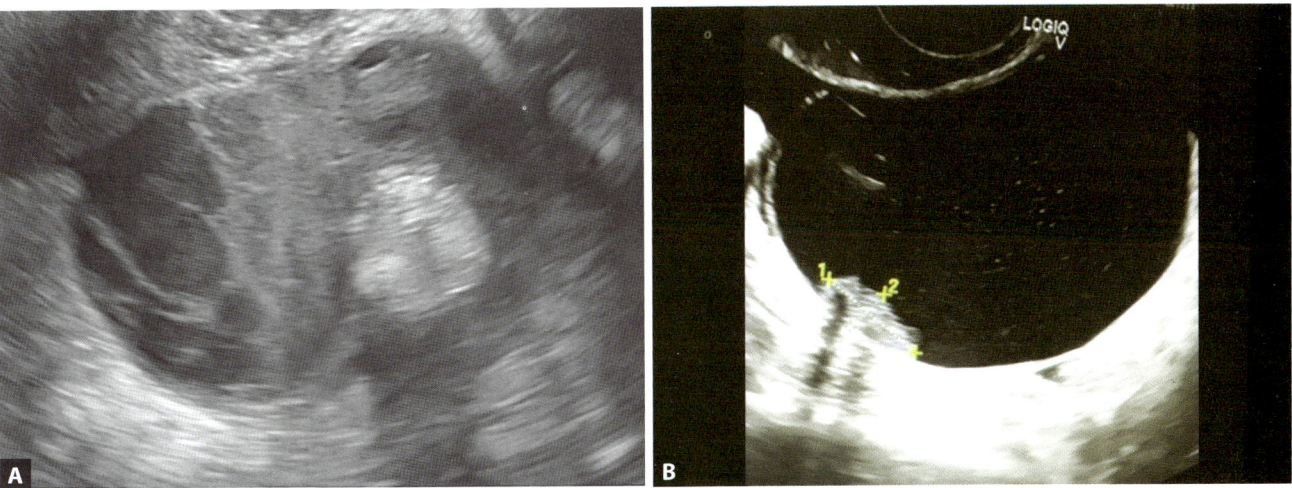

Figs. 3A and B: (A) Dermoid; (B) B. cystadenofibroma.

Flowchart 5: Differential diagnosis of intraovarian lesions of epithelial origin.

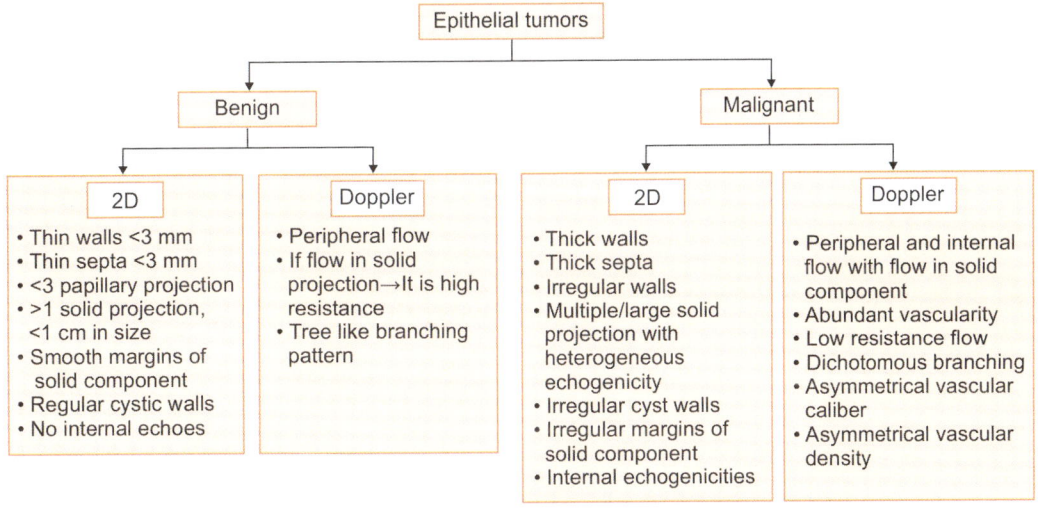

```
                        Epithelial tumors
                ┌───────────┴───────────┐
              Benign                  Malignant
          ┌─────┴─────┐           ┌─────┴─────┐
         2D         Doppler      2D         Doppler
```

Benign — 2D:
- Thin walls <3 mm
- Thin septa <3 mm
- <3 papillary projection
- >1 solid projection, <1 cm in size
- Smooth margins of solid component
- Regular cystic walls
- No internal echoes

Benign — Doppler:
- Peripheral flow
- If flow in solid projection→It is high resistance
- Tree like branching pattern

Malignant — 2D:
- Thick walls
- Thick septa
- Irregular walls
- Multiple/large solid projection with heterogeneous echogenicity
- Irregular cyst walls
- Irregular margins of solid component
- Internal echogenicities

Malignant — Doppler:
- Peripheral and internal flow with flow in solid component
- Abundant vascularity
- Low resistance flow
- Dichotomous branching
- Asymmetrical vascular caliber
- Asymmetrical vascular density

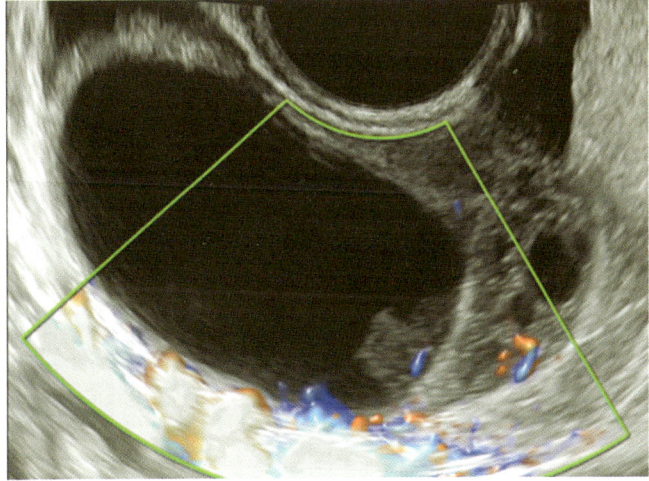

Fig. 4A

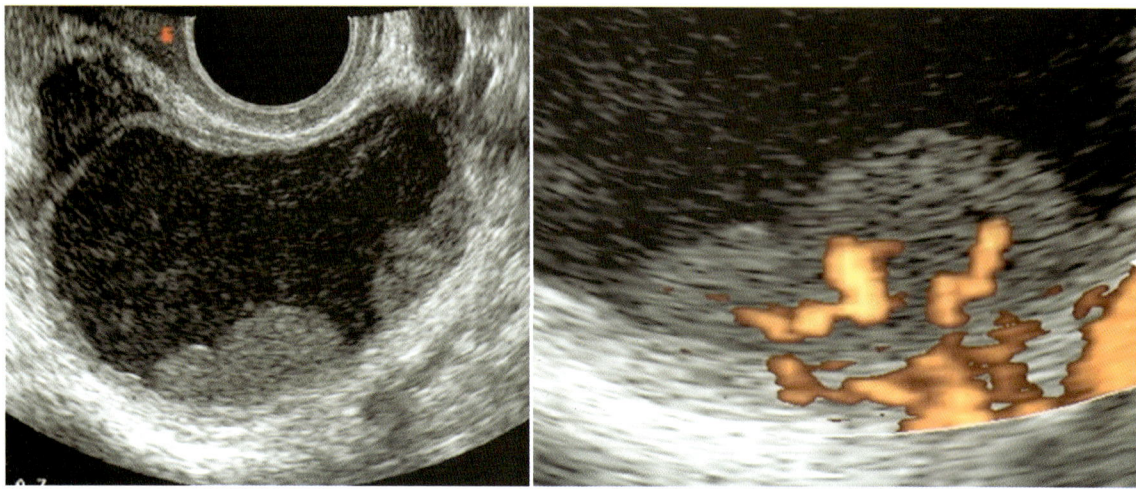

Figs. 4A and B: (A) Benign cystic lesion with solid projection; (B) Malignant benign lesion with solid projection on B mode and power Doppler.

Flowchart 6: Intraovarian cystic lesion with internal echoes.

- Hemorrhagic echogenicities (Fishnet, Honeycomb pattern, fibrin strand)
- Thick walls
- No septa
- No solid projection

Differentiate septa from fibrin strands → Rotate probe-concavity at any point of rotation—fibrin strands

Sliding sign (−) → Fixed relationship of solid component to wall of cyst
Sliding sign (+) → It is debris/clot

Corpus luteum
- In secretory phase
- Ring of color with low resistance flow on Doppler

Hemorrhagic cyst
- In proliferative phase
- No flow on Doppler
- Regresses in 3–6 weeks

Endometrioma
- May be seen in any phase of cycle

2D
- Ground glass echogenicities
- Layering effect
- Hyperechoic flecks in wall
- Hemorrhagic echogenicities

Doppler
- Short coursed vessels
- Scattered hilar vascularity

Echogenicities on 2D appearance may vary: Fishnet, Honeycomb, Fibrin strand, Isoechoic, Layering effect, Ground glass

Ground glass → Physiological in nature → CL that has stopped functioning, but has not regressed

If scanty flow:
- In proliferative phase → Regressing CL
- In secretory phase → Inadequacy of CL

Dynamic assessment → Pain on probe pressure, Adhesions

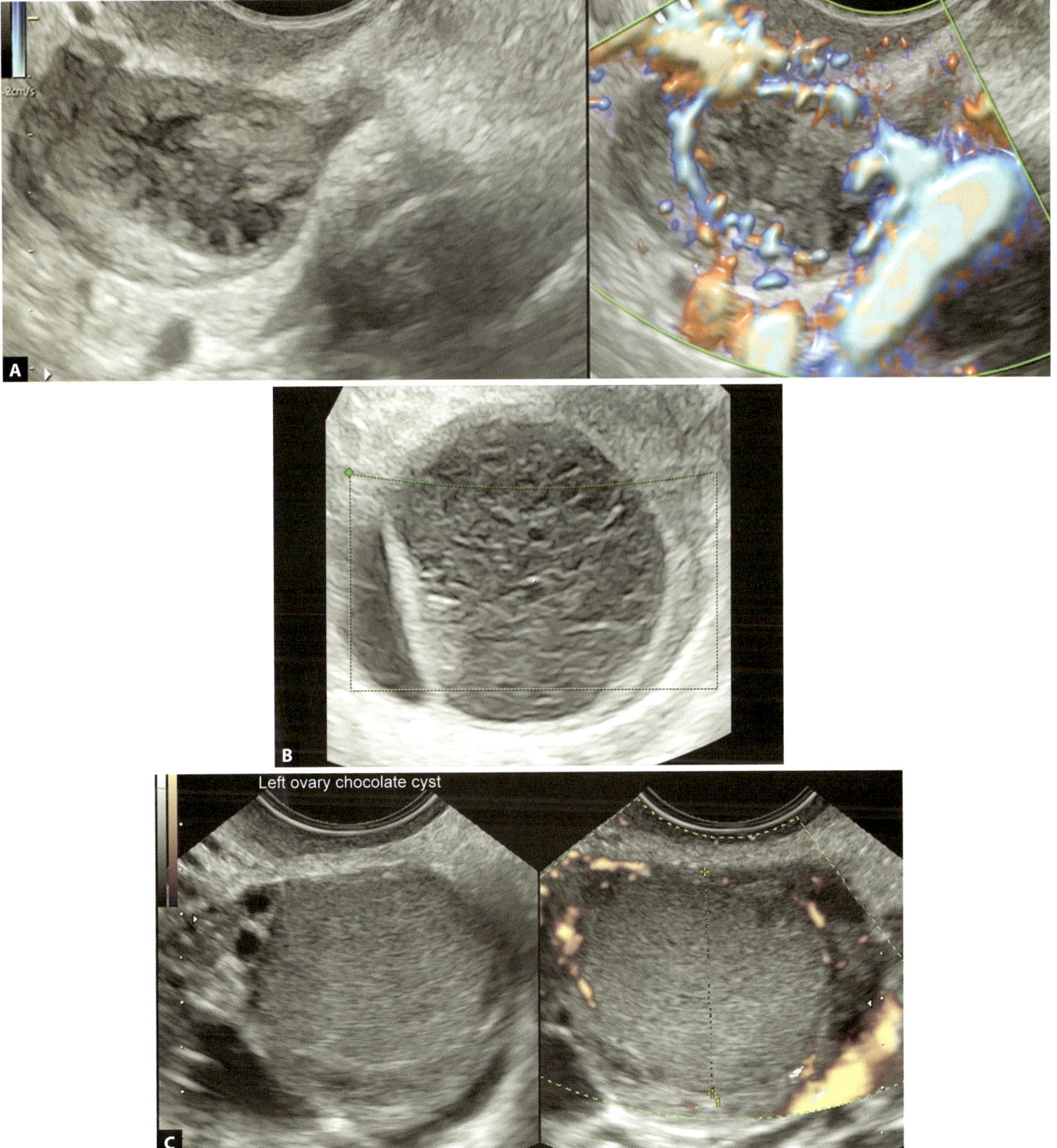

Figs. 5A to C: (A) Corpus luteum on 2D and HD flow; (B) Hemorrhagic cyst; (C) Endometrioma on B mode and power Doppler.

Chapter 17: Common Extraovarian Lesions and Pelvic Inflammatory Disease

Flowchart 1: Classification and differential diagnosis of common extraovarian lesions of pelvis.

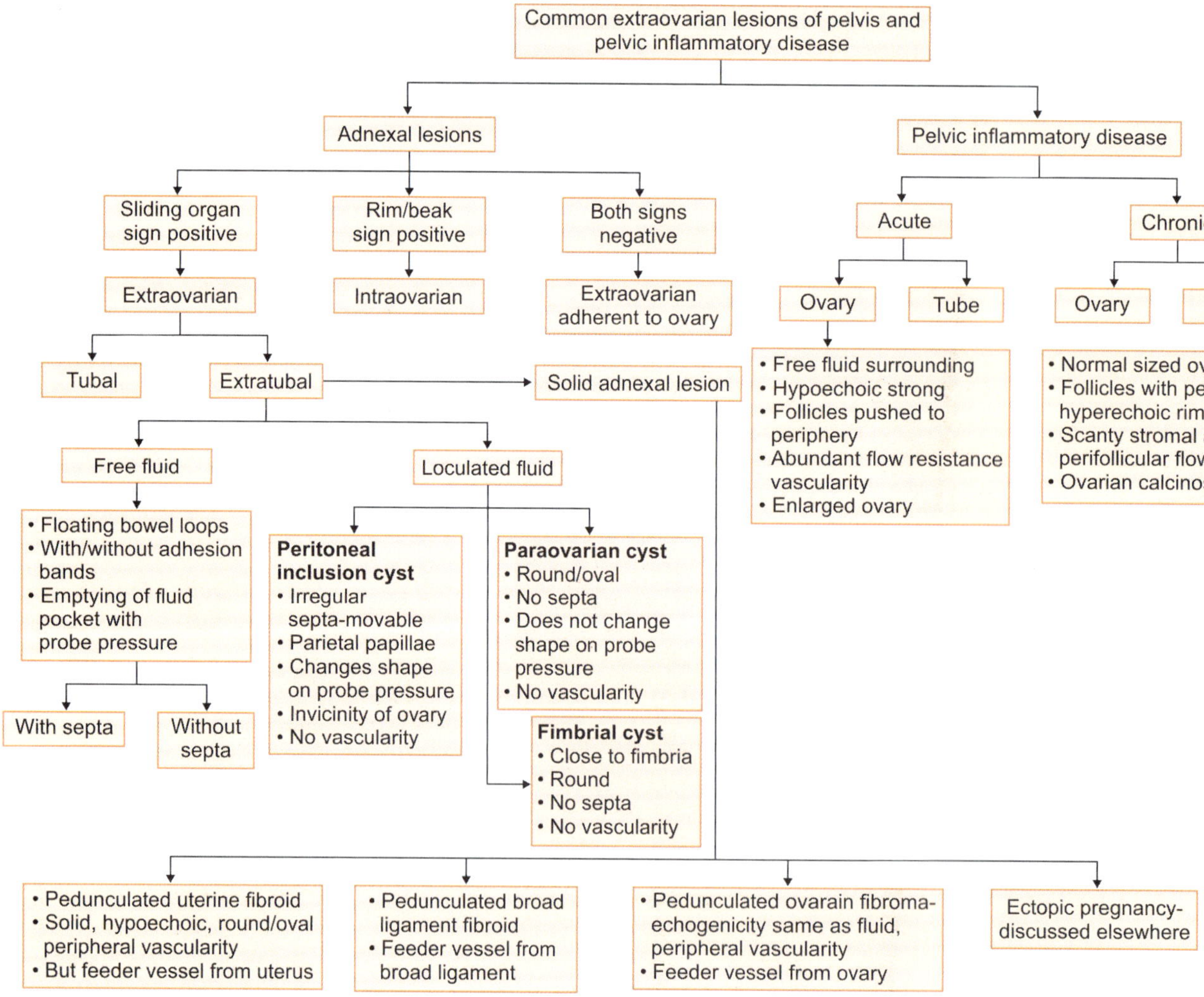

Common Extraovarian Lesions and Pelvic Inflammatory Disease 53

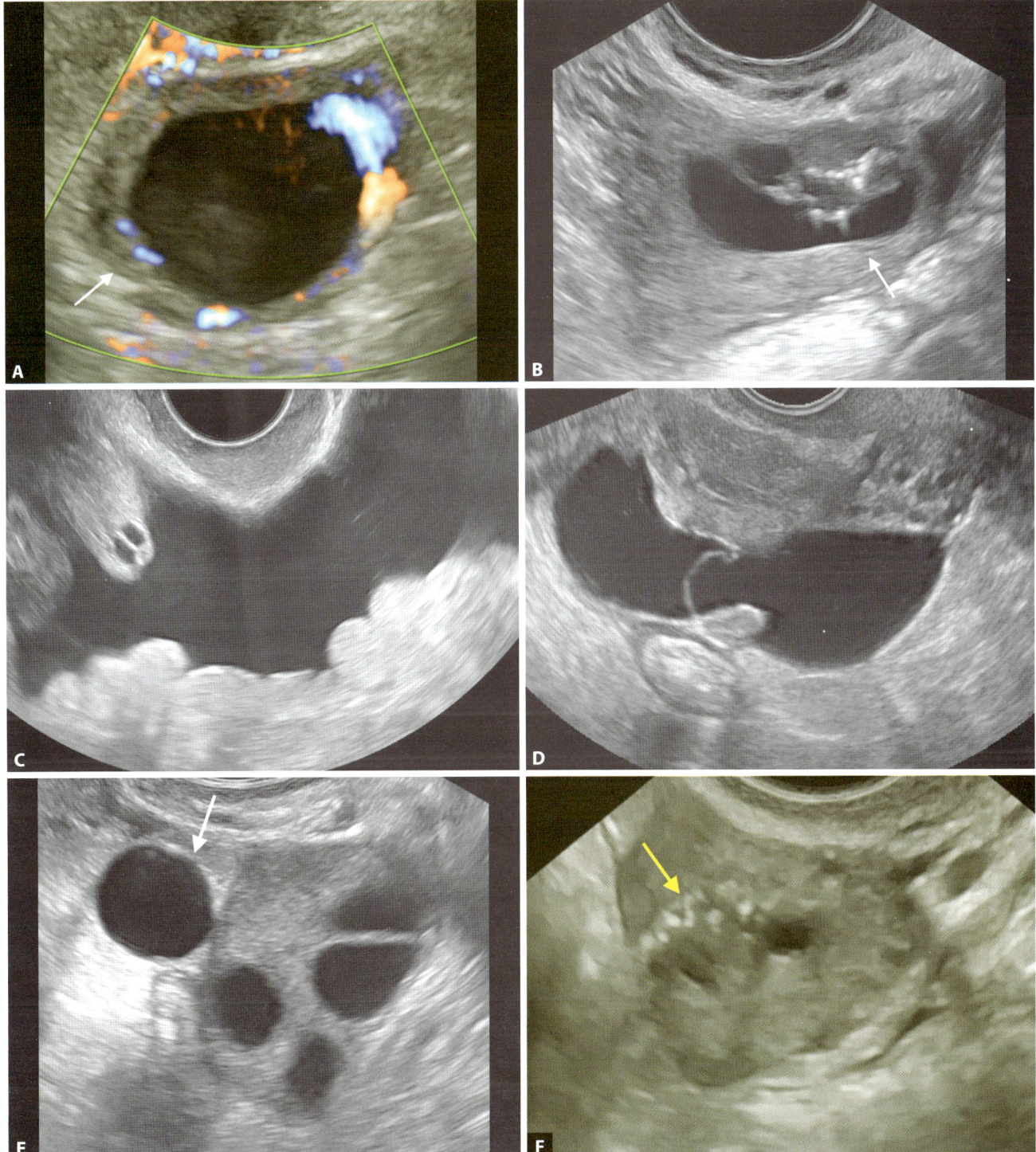

Figs. 1A to F: (A) Ovarian rim sign; (B) Ovarian beak sign; (C) Free fluid in pelvis with floating bowel loops; (D) Loculated fluid—peritoneal inclusion cyst; (E) Paraovarian cyst; (F) Ovarian calcinosis.

Common Extraovarian Lesions and Pelvic Inflammatory Disease

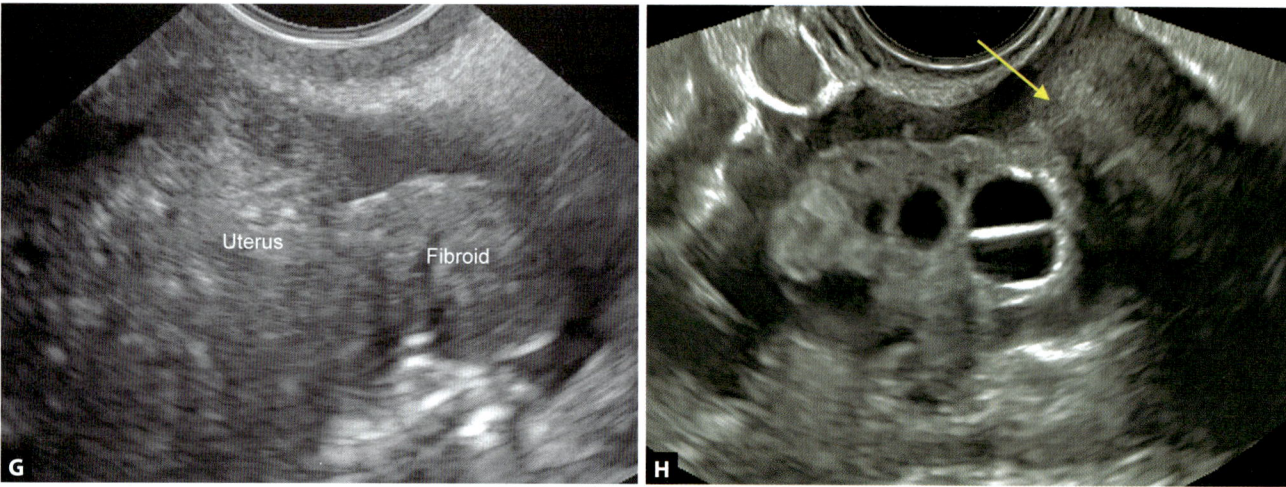

Figs. 1G and H: (G) Pedunculated uterine fibroid; (H) Pedunculated ovarian fibroma (yellow arrow).

Flowchart 2: Classification and differential diagnosis of tubal lesions.

```
Tubal lesions
├── Neoplastic
│   └── Rare
│       Ultrasound appearance same as ovarian neoplasms
│       cystic with septa, solid projections
│       vascularity depends on the type of lesion and grade of malignancy
├── Inflammatory
│   ├── Salpingitis
│   │   ├── Acute
│   │   │   • Thickened adnexal band
│   │   │   • Free fluid
│   │   │   • Increased vascularity
│   │   │   • Low resistance flow
│   │   │   • Vessels running across the width of thickened adnexal band
│   │   │   • SSG is not recommended in this stage
│   │   │   • May progress as
│   │   │       ├── Tubo-ovarian mass
│   │   │       │   • Tube and ovary adherent to each other
│   │   │       │   • With or without hydronephrosis
│   │   │       │   • Vascular score 3–4
│   │   │       └── Tubo-ovarian abscess
│   │   │           • Complex mass with solid and systic components
│   │   │           • Tube and ovary can not be identified
│   │   │           • Ovary not seen separately
│   │   │           • Vascularity varies on amount of necrosis
│   │   └── Chronic
│   │       • With or without hydrosalpinx
│   │       • Adhesions between ovary and tube even with bowel at times
│   │       • Beads on string appearance on SSG
│   └── Hydrosalpinx
│       ├── Chronic
│       │   • Thick hyperechoic walls
│       │   • Restricted lumen diameter
│       │   • At times synechiae in the tubes
│       │   • Adhesions
│       └── Acute
│           • Thick walls
│           • Solid projections on transverse section-cogwheel appearance
│           • Incomplete septa
│           • Free fluid
│           • 3D diagnostic
└── Other causes
    • Endometriosis
    • Previous surgery
```

(SSG: sonosalpingography; US: ultrasound)

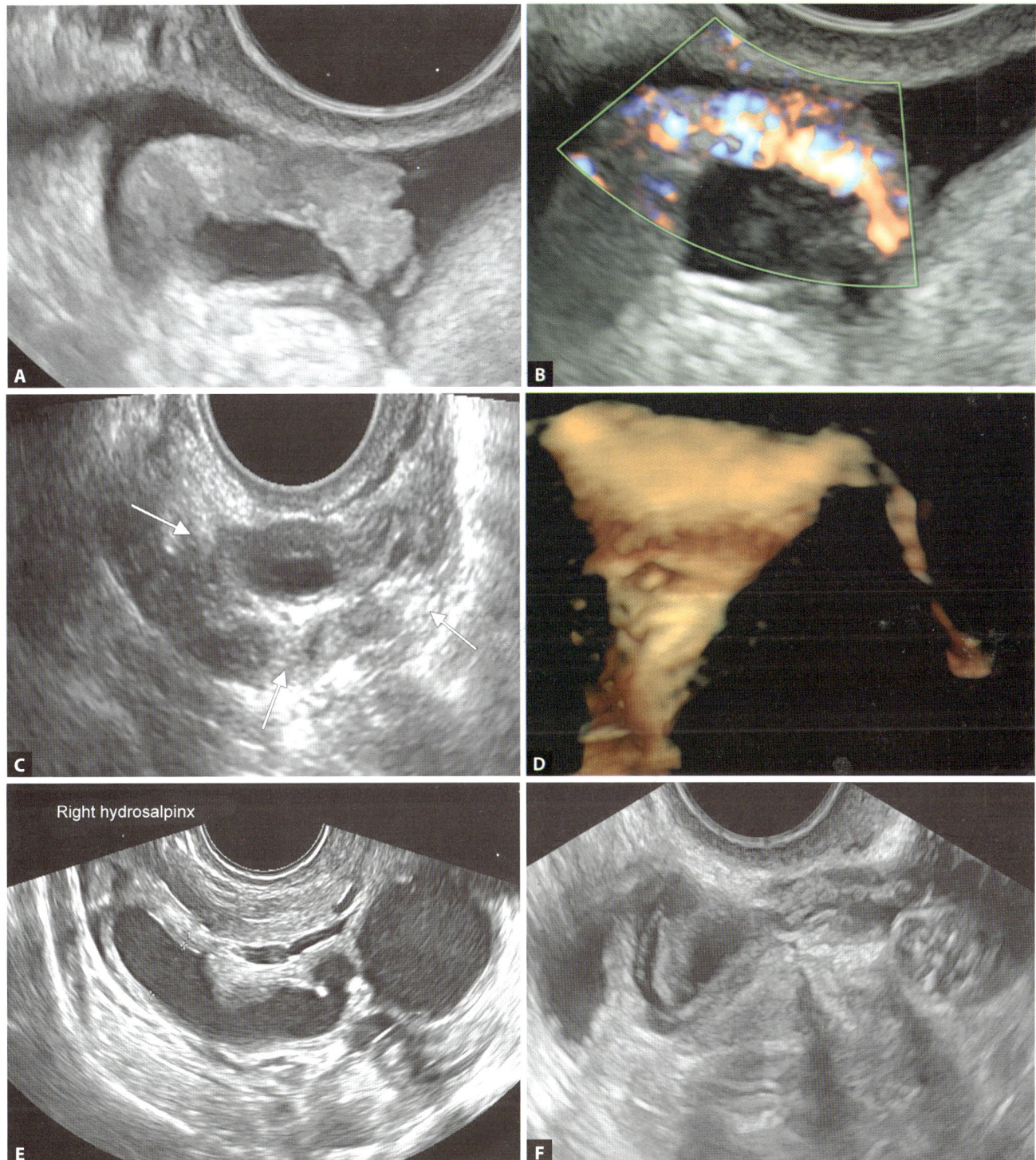

Figs. 2A to F: (A and B) B-mode and HD flow image of acute salpingitis; (C) B-mode image of chronically inflamed tube and tubo-ovarian mass (arrows); (D) 3D HyCoSy image showing beaded appearance of inflamed tube; (E) Thick walled rigid tube on B-mode with hydrosalpinx—chronic inflammatory hydrosalpinx; (F) Hydrosalpinx with thick walls—acute inflammatory hydrosalpix.

Common Extraovarian Lesions and Pelvic Inflammatory Disease

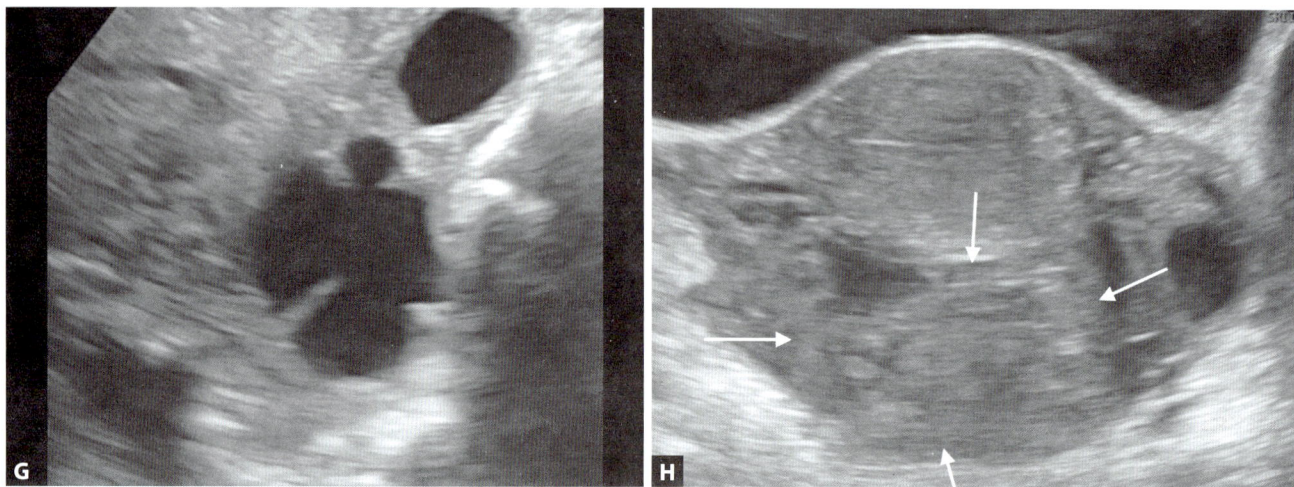

Figs. 2G and H: (G) Transverse section of acutely inflamed hydrosalpinx—cogwheel appearance; (H) Large tubo-ovarian mass seen posterior to the uterus (arrows).

Flowchart 3: Differential diagnosis of free fluid in pelvis.

```
                    Extratubal free fluid
                    /                   \
              With septa            Without septa
              /        \                  |
            PID    Preexisting adhesion   • Clear or fluid with echogenicities
             |     with fluid collection  • Common postovulatory
           Acute          |               • May also be due to high estrogen or after surgical procedure
             |     With or without        • Fibrin strands may be seen in case it is blood
    Chronic Koch's disease  echogenicities
    more common             |
             |         May be blood or pus
    • Lattice like pattern floating cysts
    • Low level echogenicities in fluid
    • Septa with nodules
```

(PID: pelvic inflammatory disease)

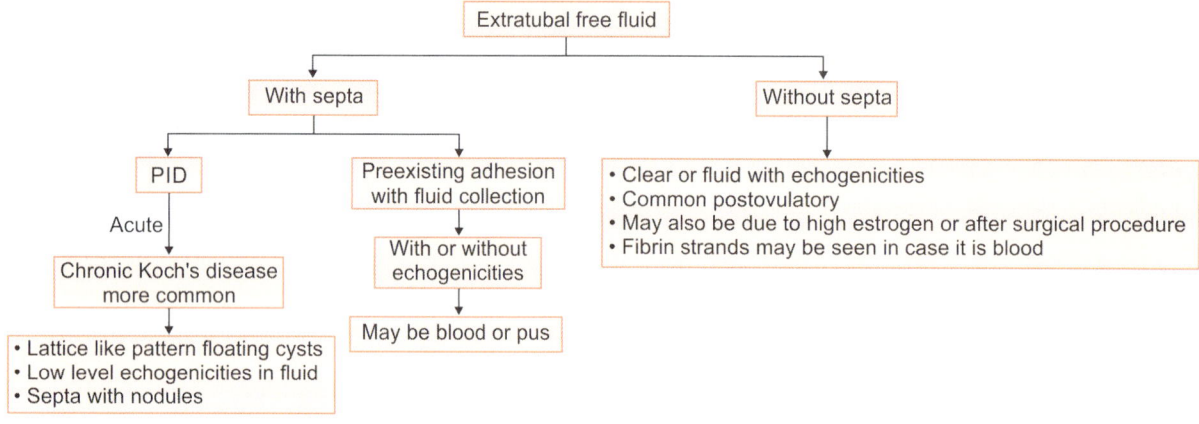

Figs. 3A and B: (A) Septated fluid collection (PID); (B) Free fluid in pelvis.

Chapter 18: Ultrasound in Gynecological Malignancies

INTRODUCTION

Gynecological malignancies refer to malignancies of uterus body–endometrium and myometrium, malignancy of cervix, ovarian malignancies, tubal malignancies, vaginal, and vulval malignancies. Though we shall also include the malignancies related to trophoblastic tissue in this chapter.

Ultrasound is the modality of choice for the assessment of the pelvic organs, and transvaginal is the preferred route for assessment of the female reproductive system. Though it is essential that the patient assessment should be started with the transabdominal scan. This allows the understanding of anatomy that may be grossly disturbed in cases of large tumors. Moreover, malignancies of reproductive organs are often associated with metastasis in peritoneum, abdominal organs, and retroperitoneal tissue, the assessment of which is not possible without an abdominal scan. Several studies have shown that using B-mode ultrasound with Doppler significantly increases the detection and diagnosis of malignancies than B-mode alone.[1] Blood vessels in malignant tumors have decreased resistance as compared to benign tumors.

The tumor vascularity develops from the host vasculature of surrounding tissues, but its organization is absolutely different from the parent vasculature. Tumor vasculature may be peripheral or central.

But whatever the distribution, the malignant vessels have some particular characteristics:[2]

- Variable caliber of the vessels
- Elongation and coiling
- Nonheirarchial vascular network, vascular rings, and sinusoids
- Abnormal precapillary architecture with dichotomous branching and no decrease in the diameter of higher-order branching
- Incomplete vascular wall with gaps in endothelium.

It is Doppler and 3D power Doppler that plays a major role in the identification of these vessel characteristics,[3] thus playing a major role in differentiating benign from malignant lesions.

Tumor vessels are dilated, saccular, and tortuous.[4] The blood in tumor vessels may flow from one venule to another venule and also through arteriovenous shunts. But only 20–80% of the vascular bed is perfused in the tumor at any particular given time.[5]

Controling the angiogenesis can serve as a complementary treatment for malignancies.[6-8] The decrease in the vascularity may occur much faster than the decrease in the size of the tumor and this can be used to assess the control of the disease.

Ultrasound contrast can be used to potentiate these Doppler signals, and it plays an important role in studying the tumor vessels and differentiating between benign and malignant tumors.[9] Volume ultrasound plays a major role in vascular studies, volume calculations, and morphological abnormalities, which may be instrumental in planning the line of treatment.

UTERINE MALIGNANCIES

Sarcoma

Sarcoma are malignant myometrial lesions found in perimenopausal patients. These consists of 1–3% of all genital tract tumors and 3–7.4% of malignant tumors of the uterine body. These lesions present like fibroids. Patients may have dysmenorrhea, menorrhagia, and pelvic pain.

On ultrasound:

- Usually single large tumor
- Hypoechoic or isoechoic but heterogenous in echogenicity with anechoic areas due to necrotic patches
- May show irregular margins, but in early stages, the margins may still be regular

- Fan shadows are not seen in these malignant tumors.
- Have a rapid growth rate
- Doppler shows peripheral vascularity with marked internal vascularity.
- Vessels have a typical chaotic pattern, with variable caliber and randomly dispersed vessels **(Fig.1)**.
- On pulsed wave Doppler, it typically shows low resistance and high-velocity flow. Like most malignant tumors the resistance index (RI) is <0.42, but even the degenerated fibroids would show heterogenous echogenicity and high internal vascularity with low resistance flow. On ultrasound, therefore, it is not possible to confidently diagnose or differentiate sarcoma from a degenerated fibroid.

Endometrial Carcinoma

Endometrial carcinoma is most common gynecological malignancy. Patients with endometrial malignancy present with menorrhagia, metrorrhagia, postmenopausal bleeding, and/or foul-smelling blood-stained vaginal discharge. The symptoms usually appear early during the disease, and therefore, these malignancies are often diagnosed early.

This tumor may have various cell types and accordingly may be classified as adenocarcinoma, papillary serous, and clear cell or mucinous carcinoma. However, 90% of the patients with endometrial malignancies have adenocarcinoma.

On ultrasound, it is not possible to confirm the histopathology.

On ultrasound:

- It is thickened on B-mode ultrasound. The endometrial thickness in literature is mentioned to be considered as suspicious of malignancy when it is >15 mm in thickness in premenopausal and >5 mm in thickness in postmenopausal age group. But it is important to mention here that if the morphology is normal and synchronous with the follicle, thickness alone cannot be considered a criterion for malignancy. Endometrial volume of >13 mL on 3D ultrasound increases the possibility of endometrial malignancy.[10]
- Heterogenous echogenicity **(Fig. 2)** may be focal or generalized.
- Anechoic areas may be seen in the endometrium, this may be due to intracavitary fluid or maybe because of blood collection in the endometrial cavity.
- Irregular endometrial surface, best appreciated on sonohysterography
- If the lesion extends toward the myometrium, the endometriomyometrial junction may appear interrupted, and the hetrogenous echogenicity may extend into the myometrium **(Fig. 3)**. Interruption of the endometriomyometrial junction has a positive likelihood ratio of 10 for endometrial malignancy. If the distance between the lower end of the mass and the external os is >2 cm, it indicates cervical invasion.

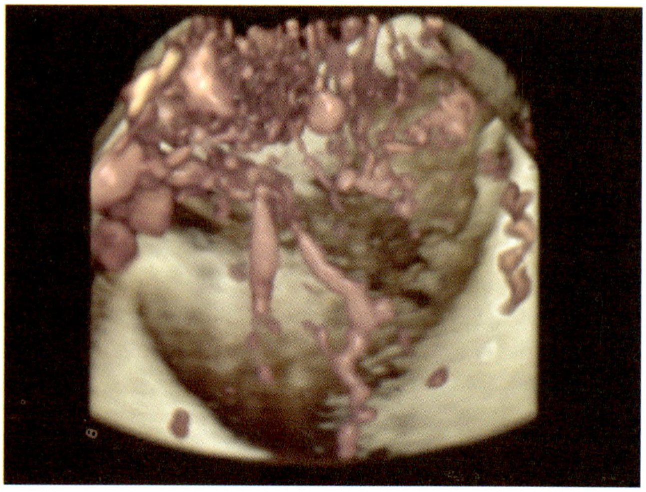

Fig. 1: Heterogenous solid lesion of the uterus with marked vascularity, with abundant branching and asymmetrical caliber suggesting the possibility of malignancy. Though theoretically, degeneration can not be excluded.

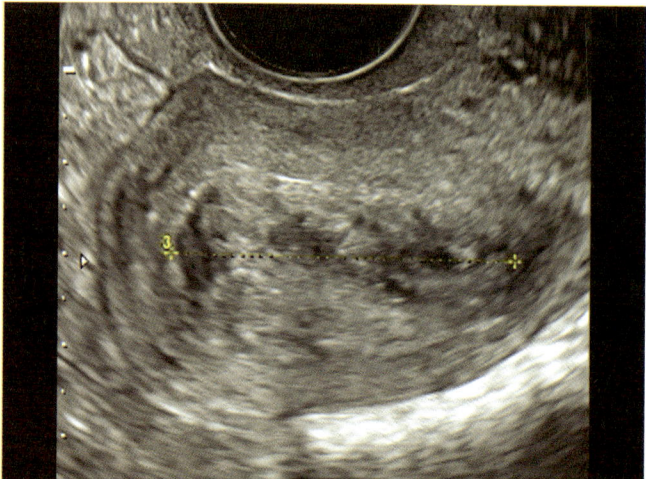

Fig. 2: Thickened endometrium with heterogenous echogenicity raising suspicion of endometrial malignancy.

Ultrasound in Gynecological Malignancies

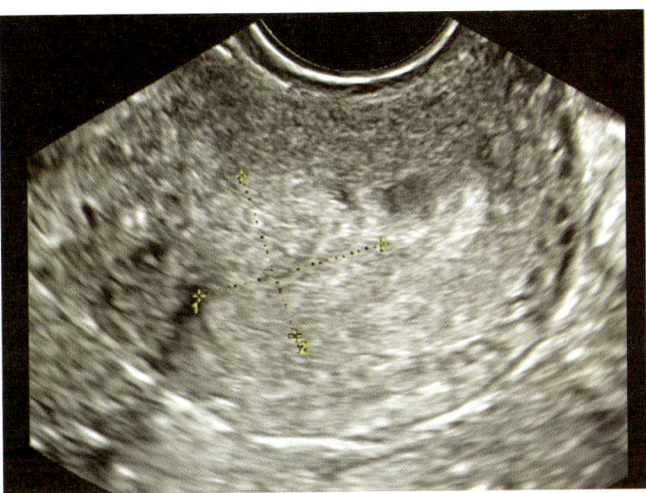

Fig. 3: Thick heterogenous endometrium with ill-defined junctional zone.

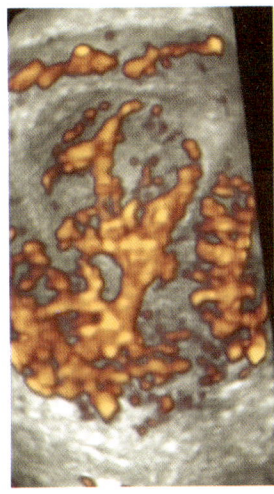

Fig. 5: 3D power Doppler of the same lesion shows abundant vascularity with abundant branching raising the suspicion of malignancy in the polyp.

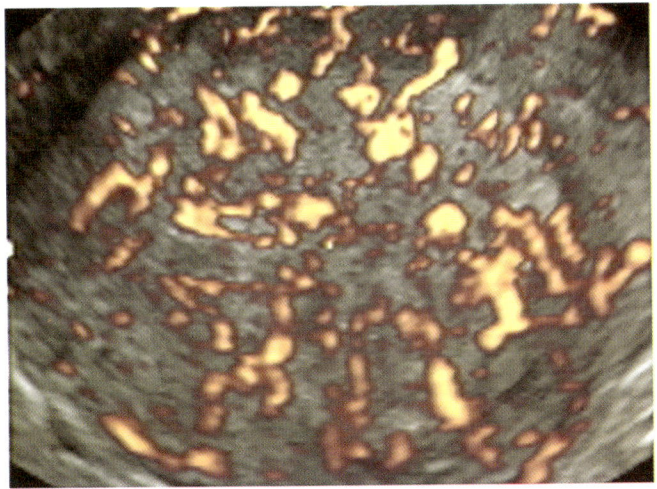

Fig. 4: Power Doppler image of the malignant mass with the vessels showing sacculations and irregular caliber.

- 3D ultrasound may be of help for better definition of the extent of the lesion by the use of volume contrast imaging (VCI) and for even more precise volume calculation by VOCAL (virtual organ computer-aided analysis).
- If the total measurement of the mass is >50% of the total uterine measurement, it indicates myometrial involvement.
- 3D ultrasound has ability to estimate the maximum penetration of the tumor in the myometrium.[11,12]
- Volume larger than 25 mL has high chance of pelvic node involvement at surgery.[13]
- Doppler studies typically show increased vascularity with low resistance flow. The vessels show sacculations and irregular caliber (Fig. 4). This vascular pattern extends with the tumor in the myometrium in case the tumor extends into the myometrium.[14]
- The vascularity is heterogeneously distributed. It is markedly increased in the growing part of the tumor and is absent in the necrotic part of the tumor.
- Vascularity score is usually 3–4. 3D power Doppler can potentially detect the lesions that require aggressive intervention. The vascularization index of endometrial carcinoma can be associated with tumor grade.[13]

Endometrial polyps may also undergo malignant change. They have:
- Irregular margins
- Heterogeneous echogenicity
- Central feeding vessel shows abundant branching with vessels showing irregular caliber and low resistance flow (Fig. 5).

Cervical Carcinoma

Cervical carcinoma is more common than endometrial carcinoma in developing countries and especially in lower socioeconomical groups. Human papilloma virus (HPV) is believed to be causative for the same. Patients with cervical carcinoma may present with intermenstrual spotting or bleeding, vaginal discharge, and may also complain of postcoital bleeding. Cervical cancer may extend into the uterine body or may extend anteriorly into bladder and posteriorly up to rectum. This may lead to symptoms like pain, melena, and hematuria.

Pap smear is an effective screening test for early diagnosis of cervical cancer. Cervical carcinoma, histologically, may be adenocarcinoma or squamous cell carcinoma.

On ultrasound:
- It may appear as isoechoic (adenocarcinoma) or hypoechoic (squamous cell carcinoma) **(Fig. 6)** solid mass lesion. Anteroposterior diameter of the cervix to the anteroposterior diameter of the corpus, normally is 0.71. If it reaches >1, it is definitely indicative of malignancy.
- Irregular margins and heterogenous echogenenicity
- When the lesions are isoechoic, these may be difficult to identify.
- Maybe endophytic or exophytic or may also be pericervical canal diamond-shaped tumors.
- Endophytic lesions are usually small and their exact location can be described by their distance from the internal os and from the cervical canal or serosa.
    - When exophytic, it is more likely to involve the surrounding structures, especially the parametrium, bladder/urethra, and rectum **(Fig. 7)**, and may lead to hydro. Large tumors may extend up to the lateral pelvic wall. Lymph gland enlargement may be seen along the iliac vessels.
- Stromal infiltration can be assessed by checking the thickness of the tumor-free cervical stroma around the margin of the tumor.
- Extension of heterogenous echogenicity in the surrounding structures and disruption of the tissue planes are seen in case of invasion. 3D ultrasound is the modality of choice for the volume assessment of the tumor mass.
    - 3D ultrasound has been used for staging of cervical carcinoma based on multiplanar imaging. Concordance of 3D ultrasound and pathology for assessing parametrial, rectal, and bladder involvement was 93%, 93% and 100%, respectively.[15]
- Vessels show irregular caliber, abundant branching, and low resistance flow **(Fig. 8)**.
- Abnormal vascular pattern is seen extending up to extension of the tumor.
- Doppler reveals four types of vascular pattern in early-stage cervical carcinomas; localized, peripheral, scattered, and single-vessel type.

Vaginal Malignancy

Vaginal malignant masses may be primary (20%) or secondary (80%). Secondaries may occur in the vagina

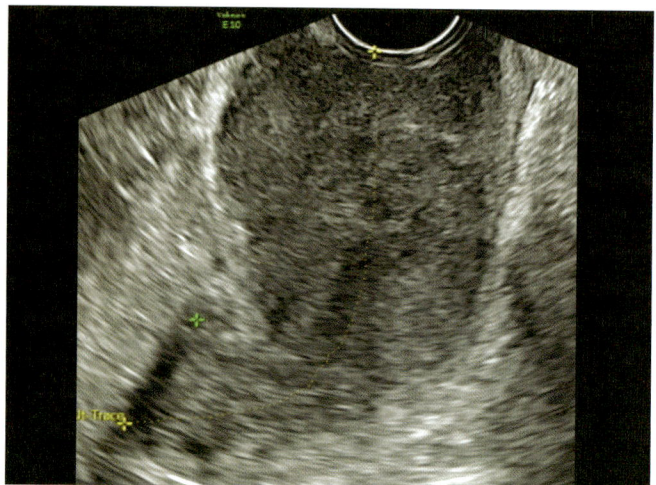

Fig. 6: B-mode image of the cervix showing marked enlargement and loss of normal anatomical planes with homogenous hypoechogenicity and a small uterine body.

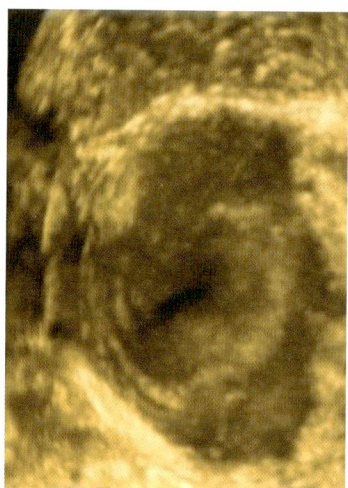

Fig. 7: A coronal plane image of the cervical maas showing irregular margins and disruption of the tissue planes. The tumor is seen extending into both parametria and also anteriorly infiltrating through the vaginal wall and posteriorly infiltrating into the rectal wall.

by local spread from cervical or vulval malignancies or by hematogenous or lymphatic spread.

Primary vaginal carcinoma: These are very rare tumors consisting of hardly 1–2% of all gynecological cancers. Histopathologically, these malignancies may be squamous cell carcinoma (most common), clear cell carcinoma, melanoma, sarcoma botryoides, and leiomyosarcoma. Patients with these tumors present with postcoital bleed, painless vaginal bleeding, vaginal discharge, and pelvic pain. If the tumor extends into bladder or bowel, the

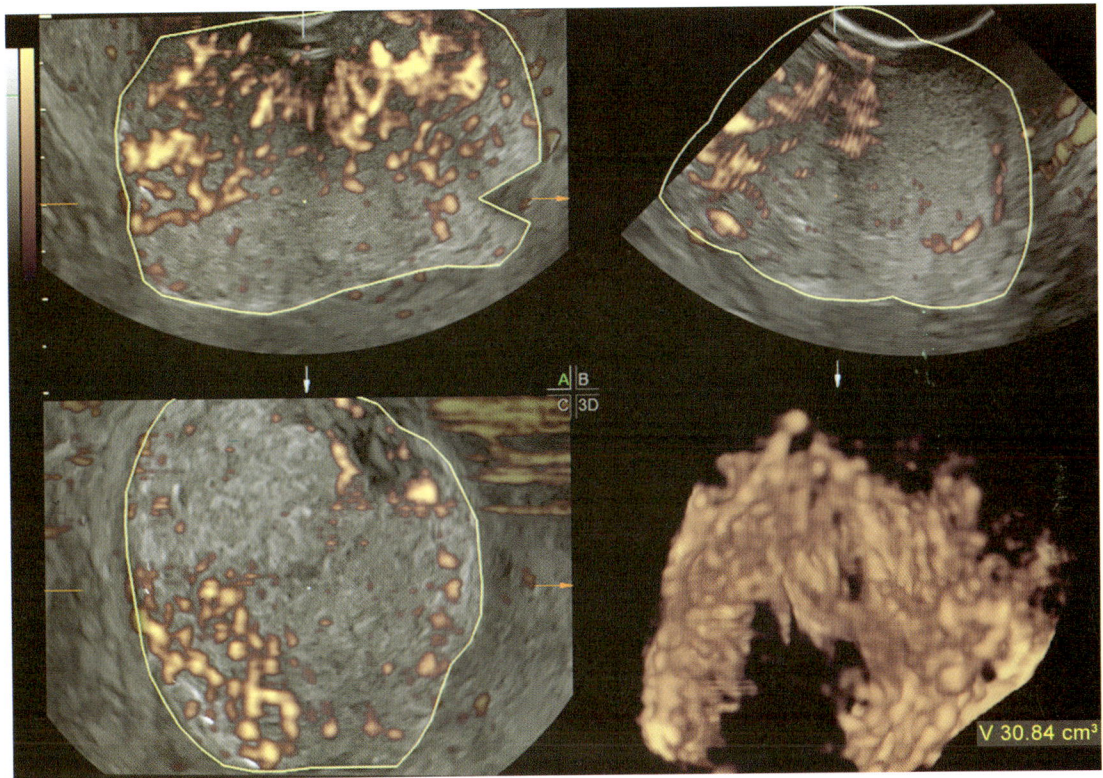

Fig. 8: 3D power Doppler image of the cervical mass showing markedly increased vascularity with vessels showing irregular caliber and abundant branching. The vascular pattern is seen extending beyond the cervix in the tumor extension.

patient may also have dysuria, hematuria, urgency, painful defecation, and constipation.

On ultrasound:
- Solid hypoechoic or heterogenous masses on transvaginal or transrectal scan
- Gel vaginosonography may improve the visibility of these lesions
- Highly vascular with score of 3–4
- Vessels are seen perpendicular to the vaginal wall
- Show irregular caliber and dichotomous branching pattern
- Extension of the hypoechoic mass in these structures and extension of the vascular pattern are also seen in these extensions.

Adnexal Lesions

Color Doppler evaluation was more accurate in the diagnosis of adnexal malignancies compared to gray scale ultrasound.[1] The vascularity was more in malignant as compared to benign tumors.[16,17] Better recognition of ovarian lesions, accurate characterization of surface features, determination of the extent of tumor infiltration, and clear depiction of the tumor volume are the advantages of 3D ultrasound.[18]

In Doppler, standardization of the power Doppler pulse repetition frequency (PRF) (0.6) and gains is essential. The sensitivity of risk of malignancy index (RMI) for ovarian malignancy was found to be 88% in one study and that for 3D power Doppler was 75% but when both were used together, showed sensitivity of 99%.[19] Another study has shown that 3D power Doppler studies had 100% positive predictive value (PPV) and 95% negative predictive value (NPV) for diagnosis of ovarian cancers.[20]

In a study by Alcazar et al.,[21] logistic regression has shown that only the central blood flow in the solid component of the tumor and ascites are independent predictors and both features correlated in 98.6% of patients of adnexal malignancy **(Box 1)**.

Contrast-enhanced 3D power Doppler has shown 100% sensitivity, 93.9% specificity, 85.7% PPV, and 100% NPV for the diagnosis of ovarian malignant lesions.

Malignant Ovarian Tumors

- *Epithelial tumors:* These may be serous, mucinous, endometrioid, clear cell, Brenner tumor and

undifferentiated tumors, and maybe borderline or malignant tumors.
- *Germ cell tumors:* Immature teratomas, dysgerminomas, yolk sac tumors, and choriocarcinoma
- *Sex cord or stromal tumors:* Granulosa cell tumor and Sertoli–Leydig cell tumor
- *Metastatic tumors*

Epithelial Tumors

- *Serous epithelial tumors:*
  - 30–50% of these may be malignant.
  - Often multilocular and maybe bilateral
  - Septa are thick and irregular.
  - May show multiple papillae and solid projections
  - Fluid part of these tumors show internal echogenicities **(Fig. 9)** may show microcalcifications or Psammoma bodies.
  - Psammoma bodies are concentric, lamellated, calcified solid components of the tumor, less echogenic than calcification and do not show acoustic shadowing.
  - Ascites may be seen.
  - On Doppler, low resistance vascularity is identified in the walls, septa, and in solid projections.
- *Mucinous epithelial tumors:* These are multilocular tumors with rigid and bright septa and internal echogenicities. Borderline tumors may show cluster of tiny locules, localized to one area **(Fig. 10)**, but tiny locules may give hyperechogenicity.

Multiple papillarities and even some solid projections may be seen **(Fig. 11)**. Low resistance flow is seen in the walls, septa, solid projections, and papillarities. Ascites with internal echogenicities may also be present.

> **BOX 1:** 3D power Doppler criteria for malignant adnexal lesions.[22]
>
> - Loss of tree-like branching pattern of vessels
> - Sacculations of arteries and veins
> - Focal narrowing of arteries
> - Internal shifts in velocity within arterial lumen
> - Beach ball finding of increased and disorganized peripheral flow around the malignant mass
> - Increased flow to center of the solid lesion
> - Crowding of vascularity
> - "Start and stop" arteries—arteries that stop abruptly without branching

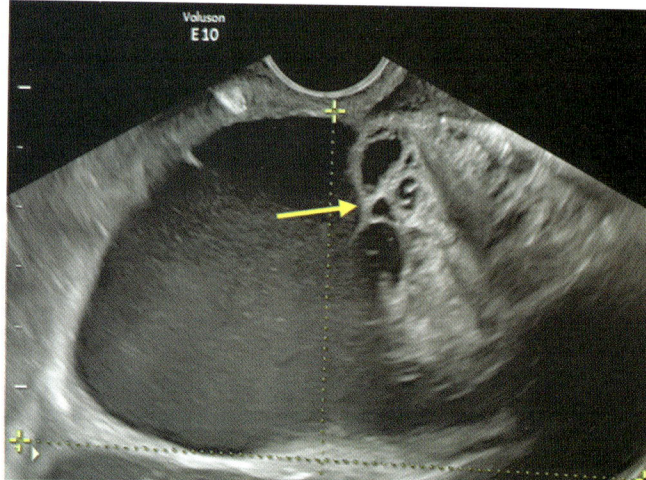

Fig. 10: Unilocular solid lesion with cluster of locules—an ultrasound appearance commonly seen in borderline tumors.

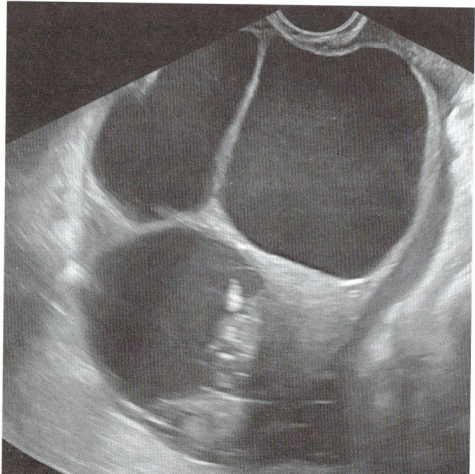

Fig. 9: B-mode ultrasound image of a multiloculated solid mass and low-level echoes in the fluid.

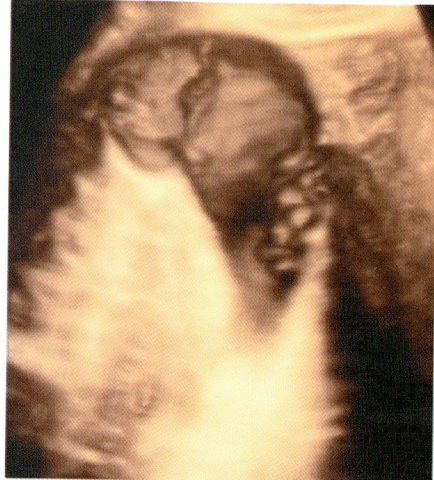

Fig. 11: 3D ultrasound image showing the solid component (multiple papillary like projections) in a unilocular cystic tumor.

Germ Cell Tumors

Malignant germ cell tumors have mixed cell types, with increased alpha-fetoprotein and human chorionic gonadotropin (hCG).

On ultrasound (in general for all germ cell tumors):
- Chiefly unilateral solid, lobulated, lesions, heterogenous echogenicity, with high-score vascularity in solid areas and septa
- Dysgerminoma is a malignant tumor of young age (second to third decade), commonly found in patients with primary amenorrhea or diagnosed during pregnancy. It maybe associated with gonadal dysgenesis of gonadoblastoma.

Sex Cord–Stromal Tumors

- *Granulosa cell tumor:* This is the most common, hormone-producing ovarian tumor; seen in postmenopausal women more commonly and in prepubertal females (5%) less commonly. These are estrogen-secreting tumors and lead to endometrial hyperplasia and occasionally endometrial carcinoma. These are large tumors with low malignant potential. On ultrasound, these appear as solid tumors with or without multiple well-defined cystic areas giving a moth-eaten appearance. The solid part of the tumor has heterogeneous echogenicity and high vascularity.
- *Sertoli and Sertoli–Leydig cell tumors (androblastomas):* These tumors of varying malignant potential, consist of Sertoli cells, Leydig cells, and fibroblasts. These tumors are more commonly seen in young women. Depending on which cell type is dominating, these may show androgenic, estrogenic, or progestogenic manifestations. These tumors also may have solid or multilocular solid appearance, with moderate-to-high vascularity.
- *Leydig cell tumor:* This is an androgen-producing tumor of postmenopausal age, typically small (mean diameter of 2.4 cm) and solid with high vascularity.

Metastatic Ovarian Tumors

Based on ultrasound features, ovarian metastatic tumors can be divided into two categories.
1. *Category A:* Solid tumors that metastasize from breast, stomach, uterus, and lymphoma.[23]
2. *Category B:* Mostly multilocular solid or multilocular tumors, but sometimes solid also, metastasized from colon, rectum, appendix, and biliary tract.

Their characteristic features include:
- Often bilateral
- Well-defined margins
- Solid/multicystic/necrotic tumors
- Solid tumors are homogeneous, unless necrosis leads to heterogenicity.
- In necrotic tumors, septa may be fragmented.
- Fluid part may be anechoic or may have low-level echoes.
- Low resistance and high-velocity flow
- "Lead vessel" with tree-like branching pattern is the typical vascular morphology of solid metastatic tumors **(Fig. 12)**.

Tubal Malignancies

Malignancy of the fallopian tubes is very rare and may comprise only about 0.18–1.6% of all gynecological malignancies. These may be difficult to differentiate from ovarian malignancies. Histopathologically, these may be serous adenocarcinoma (80%), endometrioid carcinoma, clear cell carcinoma, mucinous, or undifferentiated carcinomas. These tumors commonly occur in the distal-third of the tube and present with vaginal discharge, bleeding, abdominal pain—at times intermittent and colicky, and pelvic mass, and are more commonly found in females with a history of infertility or chronic pelvic infection.

On ultrasound:
- Solid hypo to isoechoic, with internal anechoic areas
- Ovoid or sausage-shaped mass, at times the tube may be distended with fluid

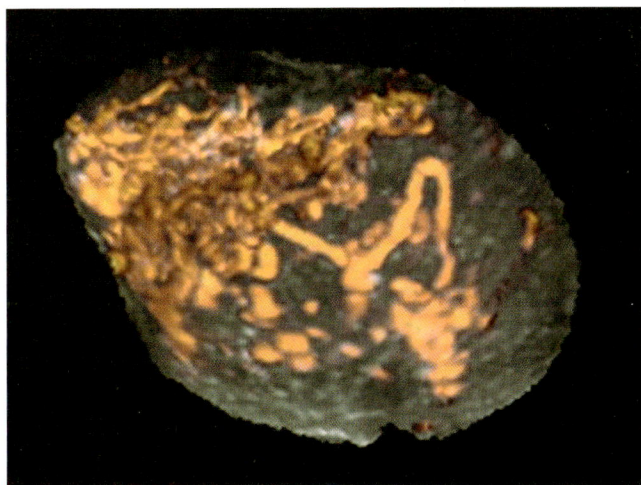

Fig. 12: 3D power Doppler ultrasound on glass body rendering showing a single feeding vessel with abundant branching and also chaotic arrangement—a metastatic ovarian tumor.

- May show mass protruding in the hydrosalpinx
- Moderate-to-high vascularity, with vessels oriented perpendicular to the mass **(Fig. 13)**.
- Free fluid may be seen in the pelvis or fluid may also be seen in the endometrial cavity.
- Ovary if seen separately, diagnosis may be more confident.

Gestational Trophoblastic Neoplasia

In patients with complete mole, the possibility of development of choriocarcinoma or invasive mole increases and this can be diagnosed by persistently high beta hCG levels after evacuation of the mole. 20% of all complete mole patients may have this risk. Though gestational trophoblastic neoplasia (GTN) may also arise after a normal pregnancy, miscarriage, or ectopic pregnancy. This group of tumors include more commonly choriocarcinoma and invasive mole and less commonly placental site trophoblastic tumor (PSTT) and epitheloid trophoblastic tumor (ETT). These may be malignant or potentially malignant. The malignant ones have a tendency to metastasize into vagina or lung. Patients present with high beta hCG levels, vaginal bleeding, hyperthyroidism, and pelvic pain. The history and clinical presentation are so typical that biopsy is usually not required for confirmation of diagnosis.

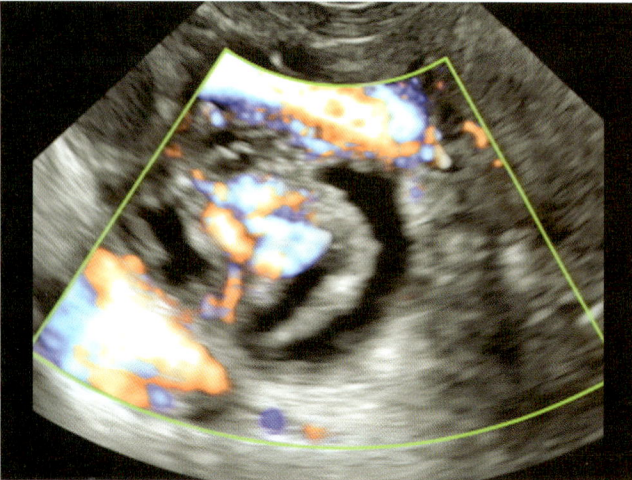

Fig. 13: Hydrosalpinx with a solid tumor seen at the center of it indicating high-definition (HD) flow showing marked vascularity in the solid part of the tumor—fallopian tube malignant tumor with hydrosalpinx.

Invasive Mole

When hydropic villi invade in the myometrium, it is called an invasive mole. On ultrasound, it appears as ill-defined solid mass in the myometrium with multiple fluid-filled anechoic areas. These lesions show high score of vascularity with low resistance flow (RI 0.4–0.45). Dilated vessels may also be seen in the surrounding myometrium. The neoangiogenesis of the mass lesion shows arteriovenous shunts, and therefore turbulent flows. Ovaries show multiloculated cystic lesions with thin septa (theca lutein cysts).

The positive response to treatment may be indicated by decreasing size and vascularity of the lesion.

Choriocarcinoma

This tumor usually follows a molar or a nonmolar pregnancy, invades in the myometrium, consists of cytotrophoblast and syncytiotrophoblast, and has a high malignant potential.

On ultrasound:

- Ill-defined solid mass with heterogenous echogenicity consisting of solid components and anechoic cystic areas secondary to hemorrhage and necrosis **(Fig. 14A)**
- Large vascular channels with moderate-to-high vascularity (score 3–4)
- Vessels of asymmetrical caliber, arteriovenous shunts, and vascular lakes **(Fig. 14B)**
- Uterine artery also shows low resistance flow.
- There maybe enlargement of the uterus heterogenicity in the myometrium.
- May extend into the parametrium
- Theca lutein cysts in ovaries with multiple loculi and thin septa

Placental Site Trophoblastic Tumor and Epitheloid Trophoblastic Tumor

These tumors arise from intermediate cells of extravillous trophoblast of nonmolar pregnancy and secrete low levels of hCG but high levels of human placental lactogen (HPL).

These tumors have indistinct margins and show multiple cystic spaces **(Fig. 15)**. The vascularity is low and the amount of vascularity represents its sensitivity to chemotherapy.

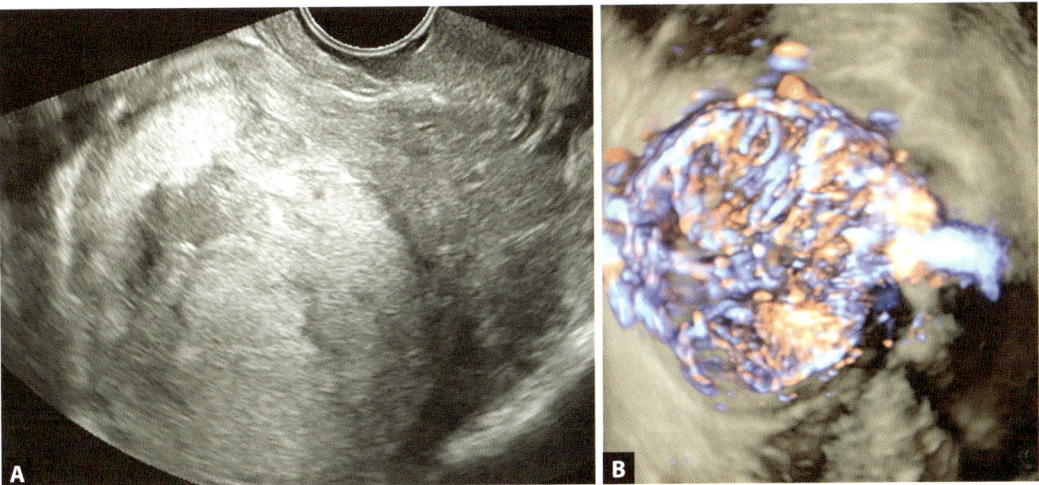

Figs. 14A and B: (A) Ill-defined solid mass lesions with heterogenous echogenicity seen on transvaginal B-mode scan; (B) Doppler shows moderate-to-high vascularity (score 3–4), with vessels of irregular caliber, arteriovenous shunts, and vascular lakes.

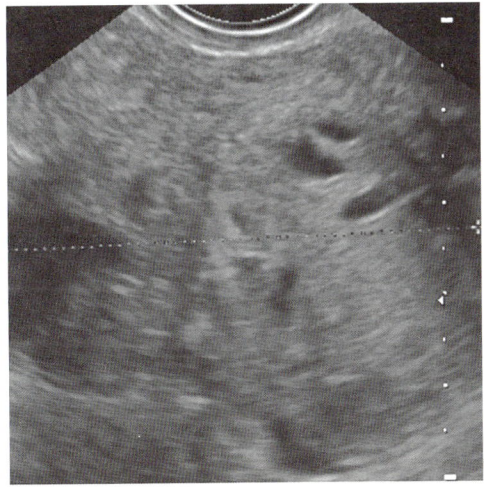

Fig. 15: Tumor with ill-defined margins and multiple small cystic spaces of variable route.

CONCLUSION

Ultrasound is a modality of choice for assessment of gynecological tumors. Transvaginal is the preferred route for more detailed assessment of these tumors. On 2D ultrasound, heterogenous echogenicity and irregular margins with extension of the lesion across the tissue planes are indicative of malignant lesion. Doppler plays an important role in assessing the vascularity of the tumor. Low resistance and high-velocity flow with vascularity score of 3–4 are the features almost consistently found in all malignancies. 3D power Doppler especially helps to study the vascular branching pattern, caliber variability, arteriovenous malformations, and venous lakes, all diagnostic of malignancy, thus increasing the sensitivity, specificity, and PPV of 3D power Doppler for diagnosis of malignant tumors.

REFERENCES

1. Kinkel K, Hricak H, Lu Y, Tsuda K, Filly RA. US characterization of ovarian masses: a meta-analysis. Radiology. 2000;217(3):803-11.
2. Kurjak A, Kupešiæ S, Breyer B. The assessment of ovarian tumor angiogenesis by three-dimensional power Doppler. In: Kurjak A (Ed). Three-Dimensional Power Doppler in Obstetrics and Gynecology. The UK: Parthenon Publishing Group; 2000.
3. Kurjak A, Kupesic S, Breyer B, Sparac V, Jukic S. The assessment of ovarian tumor angiogenesis: what does three-dimensional power Doppler add? Ultrasound Obstet Gynecol 1998,12(2):136-46.
4. Jain RK, Ward-Hartley K. Tumor blood flow: characterization, modifications and role in hyperthermia. Trans Sonics Ultrasonics. 1984;31:504-9.
5. Vaupel P, Kallinowski F, Okunieff P. Blood flow oxygen and nutrient supply, and metabolic microenvironment of human tumors: a review. Cancer Res 1989;49(23):6449-65.
6. Folkman J, Merler E, Abernathy C, Williams G. Isolation of a tumor factor responsible for angiogenesis. J Exp Med. 1971;133(2):275-88.
7. Auerbach R. Angiogenesis-inducing factors: a review. In: Pick E (Ed). Limphokines. London: Academic Press; 1981. pp. 69-88.
8. Hanahan D, Folkman J. Patterns and emerging mechanisms of the angiogenetic switch during tumorogenesis. Cell. 1996;86(3):353-64.

9. Kupešiæ S, Kurjak A. Contrast-enhanced three-dimensional power Doppler sonography for the differentiation of adnexal masses. Obstet Gynecol. 2000;96(3):452-8.
10. Gruboeck K, Jurkovic D, Lawton F, Savvas M, Tailor A, Campbell S. The diagnostic value of endometrial thickness and volume measurements by three-dimensional ultrasound in patients with postmenopausal bleeding. Ultrasound Obstet Gynecol. 1996;8:272-6.
11. Bonilla-Musoles F, Raga F, Osborne NG, Blanes J, Coelho F. Three-dimensional hysterosonography for the study of endometrial tumors: comparison with conventional transvaginal sonography, hysterosalpingography, and hysteroscopy. Gynecol Oncol. 1997;65(2):245-52.
12. Su MT, Su RM, Yue CT, Chou CY, Hsu CC, Chang FM. Three-dimesinal transvaginal ultrasound provides clearer delineation of myometrial invasion in a patient with endometrial cancer and uterine leiomyoma. Ultrasound Obstet Gynecol. 2003;22(4):434-6.
13. Saarelainen SK, Vuento MH, Kirkinen P, Mäenpää JU. Preoperative assessment of endometrial carcinoma by three-dimensional power Doppler angiography. Ultrasound Obstet Gynecol. 2012;39(4):466-72.
14. Kupešiæ S, Kurjak A, Zodan T. Staging of the endometrial carcinoma by three-dimensional power Doppler ultrasound. Gynaecol Perinatol. 1999;14:139-43.
15. Ghi T, Giunchi S, Kuleva M, Santini D, Savelli L, Formelli G, et al. Three-dimensional transvaginal sonography in local staging of cervical carcinoma: description of a novel technique and preliminary results. Ultrasound Obstet Gynecol. 2007;30(5):778-82.
16. Jokubkiene L, Sladkevicius P, Valentin L. Does three-dimensional power Doppler ultrasound help in discrimination between benign and malignant ovarian masses? Ultrasound Obstet Gynecol. 2007;29(2):215-25.
17. Kudla MJ, Timor-Tritsch IE, Hope JM, Monteagudo A, Poiolek D, Monda S, et al. Spherical tissue sampling in 3-dimensional power Doppler angiography: a new approach for evaluation of ovarian tumors. J Ultrasound Med. 2008;27(3):425-33.
18. Riccabona M, Nelson TR, Pretorius DH. Three-dimensional ultrasound: accuracy of distance and volume measurements. Ultrasound Obstet Gynecol 1996;7(6):429-34.
19. Mansour GM, El-Lamie IK, El-Sayed HM, Ibrahim AM, Laban M, Abou-Louz SK. Adnexal mass vascularity assessed by three-dimensional power Doppler: does it add to the risk of malignancy index in prediction of ovarian malignancy? Four hundred-case study. Int J Gynecol Cancer 2009;19(5):867-72.
20. Chase DM, Crade M, Basu T, Saffari B, Berman ML. Preoperative diagnosis of ovarian malignancy: preliminary results of the use of three-dimensional vascular ultrasound. Int J Gynecol Cancer. 2009;19(3):354-60.
21. Alcazar JL, Royo P, Pineda L, Ruiz-Zambrana, Auba M, Olartecoechea B. Which parameters could be useful for predicting malignancy in solid adnexal masses? Donald School Journal of Ultrasound in Obstetrics and Gynecology 2009;3(1): 1-5.
22. Crade M. Tissue block ultrasound and ovarian cancer- a pictorial presentation of findings. DSJUOG. 2009;3(1):41-7.
23. Testa AC, Ferrandina G, Timmerman D, Savelli L, Ludovisi M, Van Holsbeke C, et al. Imaging in gynecological disease (1): Ultrasound features of metastases in the ovaries differ depending on the origin of the primary tumor. Ultrasound Obstet Gynecol. 2007;29(5):505-11.

Chapter 19: Ultrasound for Diagnosis of Endometriosis

INTRODUCTION

By definition, endometriosis when extends to >5 mm deep from the peritoneal surface, is named deep-infiltrating endometriosis (DIE). But according to the new definition (2021), deep endometriosis is endometriosis that is not on the peritoneum and not necessarily infiltrating.[1] DIE may involve bowel, bladder, uterosacral ligament, and vaginorectal septum, most commonly, but may also involve abdominal organs at times. DIE presents as dysmenorrhea, dyspareunia, chronic pelvic pain, and often dysuria or pain on defecation, apart from infertility. The endometriotic patch typically leads to invasion, inflammation, myoproliferation, and fibrosis, leading to distortion of surrounding anatomy. It is seen in 4–13% of women in reproductive age group and in 25–50% of women with infertility.

On ultrasound **(Flowchart 1)**:

- These lesions generally appear as ill-defined irregular hypoechoic areas with or without acoustic shadowing.
- These lesions typically show hyperechoic spots due to hemosiderin and cholesterol deposits.

Flowchart 1: Ultrasound in endometriosis.

```
                              Ultrasound in endometriosis
    ┌──────────────────┬───────────────────┬──────────────────────┬────────────────────┐
Detailed ultrasound   Soft markers like    Deep endometriosis      Superficial endometriosis
of uterus, ovary,     sliding organ sign   ┌──────────┬─────────┐  • Can be diagnosed in
and adnexa            tenderness guided US Posterior   Anterior    presence of free fluid
        │                                  compartment compartment • Floating tissue tags
Discussed in                               assessment  assessment  • Floating hyperechoic
dedicated chapters                                                   flecks from the
                                                                     peritoneum, or
                                                                     uterine wall
                                                                   • Hat-like hypoechoic
                                                                     areas and hypoechoic
                                                                     nodules
                                                                   • Pain on probe pressure
```

Posterior compartment assessment branches into:

- **Uterosacral ligament (USL)**: Slide the probe gently into posterior fornix. Identify posterior vaginal wall and overlying thin hyperechoic peritoneum in sagittal plane. Rotate probe and slide laterally to observe thickening and splaying of this hyperechoic line laterally (USL).
  - Hat-like hypoechoic lesions
  - Hyperechoic margins
  - Hypoechoic nodules
  - Scattered vascularity
  - Pain on probe pressure

- **Rectovaginal septum where vagina and rectum are in close apposition**:
  - Identify tissue layers
  - Discontinuity or irregularity in these layers
  - Hypoechoic lesion distorting these tissue layers with irregular margins, hyperechoic flecks, peripheral hyperechoic margins, projection like extensions in surrounding tissue plane, adhesions

- **Bowel endometriosis trace anterior muscularis**: Broadening of hypoechoic muscularis with irregular hypoechoic lesion with finger like extensions due to adhesions, hyperechoic peripheral area due to myoproliferation, adhesions-absent, sliding sign, pain on probe pressure, hyperechoic flecks in lesion

Anterior compartment assessment: Focal outer adenomyotic nodule on posterior wall of uterus — Hypoechoic illdefined irregular margin with hyperechoic lines and dots may/may not be adherent to bowel pain on probe pressure

(US: ultrasound)

- These are tender on probe pressure.
- Typically hypovascular
- Adhesions of involved surfaces are common.
- Transvaginal scan has shown 81.1% sensitivity and 94.2% specificity for diagnosis of DIE.[2]
- Transrectal scan can especially be of help in patients with involvement of the posterior compartment endometriosis.

SYSTEMATIC ASSESSMENT

According to International Deep Endometriosis Analysis (IDEA) consensus:
- Detailed assessment of the uterus, ovaries, and adnexa
- Tenderness-guided ultrasound
- Assessment for sliding organ sign to rule out adhesions
- *Posterior compartment assessment:* Slide the probe through the introitus with posterior angulation to follow the anterior muscularis of the bowel and the interface between the posterior vaginal wall. Sliding of the bowel on the vaginal wall is assessed.
- *Anterior compartment assessment:* Slide the probe into the anterior fornix to assess the posterior muscularis of the urethra and interface between the posterior urethral wall, posterior bladder wall, and the vagina.

RECTOSIGMOID DEEP-INFILTRATING ENDOMETRIOSIS

The characteristics of rectosigmoid DIE are:
- It usually involves the anterior muscularis of the rectosigmoid part of the large bowel.
- Discontinuity of the line that is seen in the middle of muscularis layer, separating longitudinal and circular muscle layer, due to a fusiform or elongated hypoechoic area indicates endometriosis **(Fig. 1)**.
- On transverse section, this typically gives a signet ring appearance.
- If submucosa is involved, fibrotic retraction of the lesion in the submucosa leads to a typical "Red Indian head" appearance.
- Negative sliding organ sign between the uterus and the bowel may be an additional sign and has a likelihood ratio of 23.6 for rectal DIE.[3]

VAGINAL DEEP-INFILTRATING ENDOMETRIOSIS

- Localized hypoechoic thickening of the vaginal wall, without well-defined margins
- Vaginal wall thickening can be more clearly appreciated with gel vaginosonography.

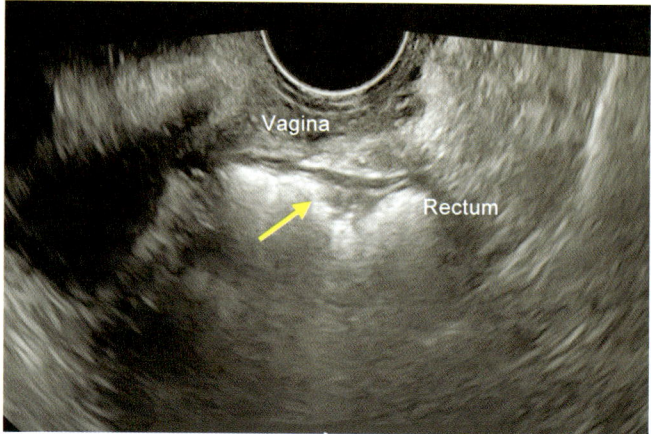

Fig. 1: Rectovaginal endometriotic patch shown by the yellow arrow in 2D ultrasound image.

CERVICAL DEEP-INFILTRATING ENDOMETRIOSIS

- Thick, firm cervical wall with hypoechoic area on ultrasound with ill-defined margins
- Lesions are tender on probe pressure.

UTEROSACRAL DEEP-INFILTRATING ENDOMETRIOSIS

The characteristics of uterosacral DIE **(Fig. 2)** are as follows:
- Uterosacral ligament is seen as a thick soft-tissue mass posterior to the uterus and extending to bowel.
- Placing the probe deep in the posterior fornix in longitudinal plane, with downward angulation will show isoechoic posterior vaginal wall and posterior to it a thin hyperechoic line—peritoneum. Rotate the probe anticlockwise and span it laterally tracing the peritoneal shadow. This hyperechoic line of peritoneum gradually thickens and then splays a little laterally as hyperechoic band. This is uterosacral ligament.
- Hypoechoic lesion (hat-like) with irregular margins in the thickened uterosacral ligament, hypoechoic nodules, and hyperechoic flecks in the uterosacral ligament
- Tender on probe pressure

DEEP-INFILTRATING ENDOMETRIOSIS IN THE BLADDER

- Localized thickening of bladder wall, hypoechoic, and hypovascular on ultrasound. These may sometimes appear like localized solid projections.

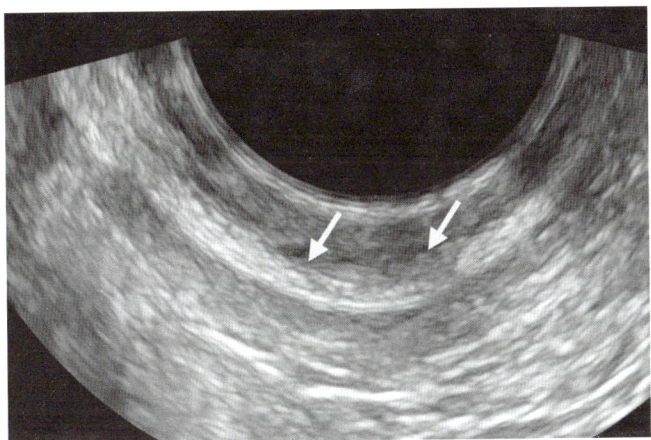

Fig. 2: Hypoechoic lesion (hat-like) with irregular margins in the thickened uterosacral ligament, hypoechoic nodules, and hyperechoic flecks in the uterosacral ligament (White arrows).

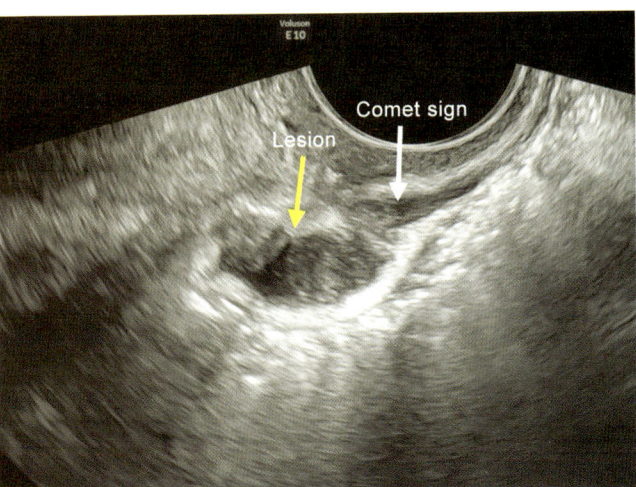

Fig. 3: Typical bowel endometriosis.

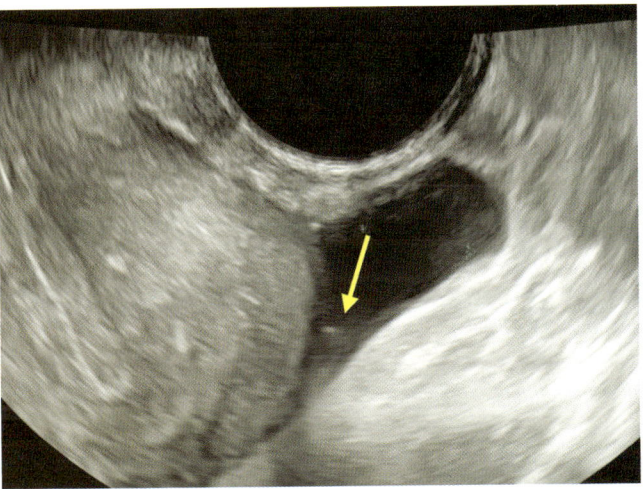

Fig. 4: Superficial endometriosis (yellow arrow).

- Trigone is the area most commonly affected
- If it may involve the bladder diffusely, it gives a typical hourglass shape to the bladder. When in bladder, it may also involve the ureteric insertion and may lead to obstruction and hydronephrosis.
- Check the sliding of the bladder on the uterus.
- Involvement of ureters is to be checked. (The intravesical segment of the ureter is identified and its course is followed to where it leaves the bladder and then further, to the pelvic side wall and up to the level of the bifurcation of the common iliac vessels.)
- More common on bladder base and bladder dome.

For ease of reporting, the bladder is divided into four zones:
1. *Trigone:* Within 3 cm of urethral opening
2. *Bladder base:* Faces backward and downward adjacent to both the vagina and the supravaginal cervix
3. *Bladder dome:* Intraabdominal and superior to bladder base
4. Extra-abdominal bladder

Endometriotic lesions **(Fig. 3):**
- May affect muscularis or mucosa
- Only serosal involvement is superficial and difficult to diagnose.
- Hypoechoic linear or spherical lesions
- Three longest orthogonal diameters
- Confirm adhesions between bladder and uterus, but need to remember that adhesions may also be due to previous cesarean section or any other surgery.

SUPERFICIAL ENDOMETRIOSIS

Superficial endometriosis may be seen anywhere in the pelvis and also at times in the abdominal cavity, but the most common are ovarian and uterine surfaces, peritoneum, and uterosacral ligaments.

It is suspected in the presence of minimal fluid and floating flimsy solid projections or septa-like echogenic lesions that move on probe movement. Sometimes it is also seen as tiny echogenic flecks floating from the surface of peritoneum or organ. It may also be seen as tiny hypoechoic deposits **(Fig. 4)**.

SonoPODgraphy with 20–30 mL of saline injection through cervix into the pouch of Douglas can lead to a better demonstration of the lesion.

In case of retroverted uterus, gentle probe movement in and out can lead to a collection of triangular pocket of fluid posterior to the uterus, between uterus and cervix, this is a sign of free mobility and no adhesions, and therefore no endometriosis in that region. Inability to do this and the feeling of a thick nodule or inability to further slide the probe in this direction indicates endometriosis.

CONCLUSION

Ultrasound plays a major role in the diagnosis of endometriosis, especially for laparoscopically inaccessible areas. It can give comparable results to magnetic resonance imaging (MRI) for the same but being an operator-dependent modality, its efficacy may vary according to the expertise of the operator.

REFERENCES

1. International Working Group of AAGL, ESGE, ESHRE, and WES; Tomassetti C, Johnson NP, Petrozza J, Abrao MS, Einarsson JI, Horne AW, et al. An international terminology for endometriosis, 2021. Hum Reprod Open. 2021;2021(4):hoab029.
2. Vimercati A, Achilarre MT, Scardapane A, Lorusso F, Ceci O, Mangiatordi G, et al. Accuracy of transvaginal sonography and contrast-enhanced magnetic resonance colonography for presurgical staging of deep infiltrating endometriosis. Ultrasound Obstet Gynecol. 2012;40(5):593-603.
3. Hudelist G, Fritzer N, Staettner S, Tammaa A, Tinelli A, Sparic R, et al. Uterine sliding sign: a simple sonographic predictor for presence of deep infiltrating endometriosis of the rectum. Ultrasound Obstet Gynecol. 2013;41(6):692-5.

Baseline Scan

INTRODUCTION

Success of any assisted reproductive technology is chiefly dependent on two decisions, selection of correct stimulation protocol and correct timing of ovulation trigger. Selection of correct stimulation protocol is based on prestimulation assessment of female to assess ovarian response and reserve. This is done by baseline ultrasound scan on 2nd–3rd day of menstrual cycle **(Flowchart 1)**. At this period of menstrual cycle, the ovarian steroids and pituitary hormones are all at their baseline level. Ovaries must have no active follicle or corpus luteum at this stage to satisfy this hormonal status.

WHAT TO SEE?
Antral Follicle Count and Ovarian Volume

To assess ovarian reserve (How many follicles can be grown?)

Antral follicle count (AFC) is the most useful marker in predicting ovarian response. Doing AFC assessment alone would be more cost-effective for predicting the ovarian reserve in patients undergoing controlled ovarian stimulation with gonadotropin hormone-releasing hormone (GnRH) antagonist. AFC had the highest accuracy for predicting ovarian reserve in patients with abnormal ovarian reserve test and was statistically significant (number of oocytes aspirated p-value <0.001) than anti-Müllerian hormone (AMH) (p-value 0.06) and follicle-stimulating hormone (FSH) (p-value 0.212) in predicting ovarian reserve.

For the prediction of poor ovarian reserve, a model including AFC + AMH was found to be almost similar to that of (p-value 0.001) using AFC alone.[1]

Precise calculation of AFC, therefore, can help in predicting the ovarian reserve.

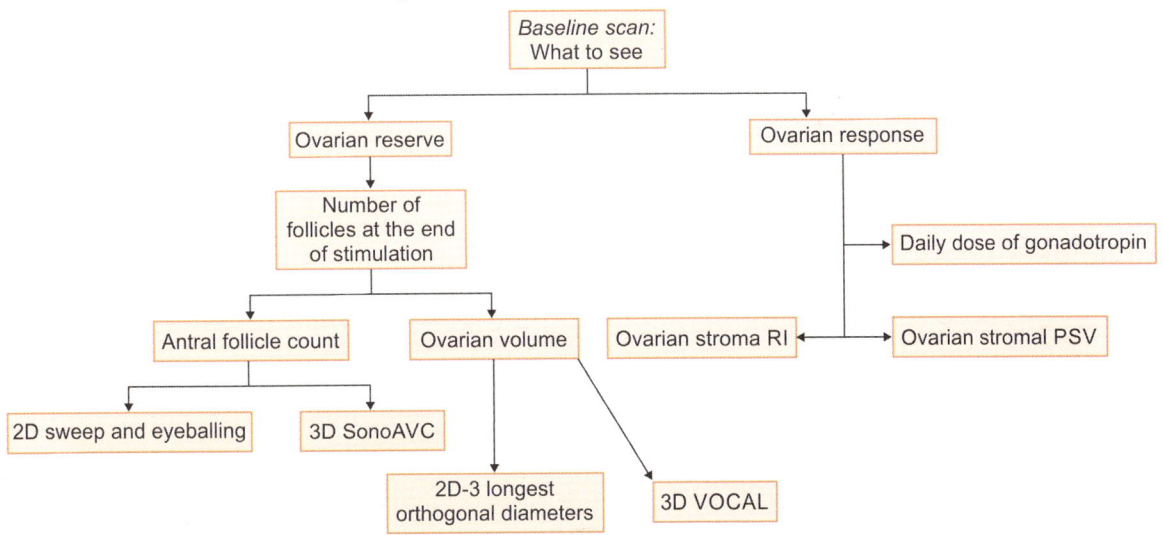

Flowchart 1: Algorithm to be followed for baseline scan (day 2 scan).

(PSV: peak systolic velocity; RI: resistance index; SonoAVC: sonography-based automated volume count; VOCAL: virtual organ computer-aided analysis)

How to count antral follicles?
2D ultrasound: Scroll across the ovary and eyeball to count. Do not rotate the probe or sweep the probe back.

3D with sonography-based automated volume count (SonoAVC): This is a specialized 3D ultrasound software for the calculation of antral follicle number and volume. This method is more precise when follicles are multiple [>15 follicle number per ovary (FNPO)]. But postprocessing is required for accurate calculations **(Fig. 1)**.

Freiesleben et al. concluded that body weight and AFC may be used to achieve appropriate assessment of ovarian reserve for intrauterine insemination (IUI) in ovulatory patients.[2]

Ovarian volume was also used in decision-making for stimulation protocol for ovarian induction. Ovarian volume correlates with number of oocytes retrieved.[3]

Ovarian volume <3 cm^3 was significantly predictive of higher in vitro fertilization (IVF) cancellation rates (>50%).[4] Ovarian volume can be calculated by measuring three longest orthogonal diameters of the ovary or by the 3D software virtual organ computer-aided analysis (VOCAL). The latter is more reliable when the ovary is not round or oval **(Fig. 2)**.

Ovarian volume and AFC correlate to the number of follicles matured and oocytes retrieved.[5] AFC and ovarian volume provide direct measurements of ovarian reserve.[6]

Ovarian Stromal Flow

To assess ovarian response and dose of gonadotropins

Measurement of ovarian stromal flow in early follicular phase is related to subsequent ovarian response in IVF treatment **(Fig. 3)**.[7] Ovarian stromal peak systolic velocity (PSV) after pituitary suppression is predictive of ovarian responsiveness and outcome of IVF treatment.[8] Ovarian blood flow predicts ovarian responsiveness and hence provides a noninvasive and cost-effective prognostic factor of IVF outcome.[9]

Measuring ovarian stromal flow: Locate the ovary and switch on the color Doppler box. Adjust its size so that it includes the entire ovary. Pulse repetition frequency (PRF) is set at 0.3 and the wall motion filter (WMF) is set at the lowest. As the vessels are seen in the ovary, gently scroll

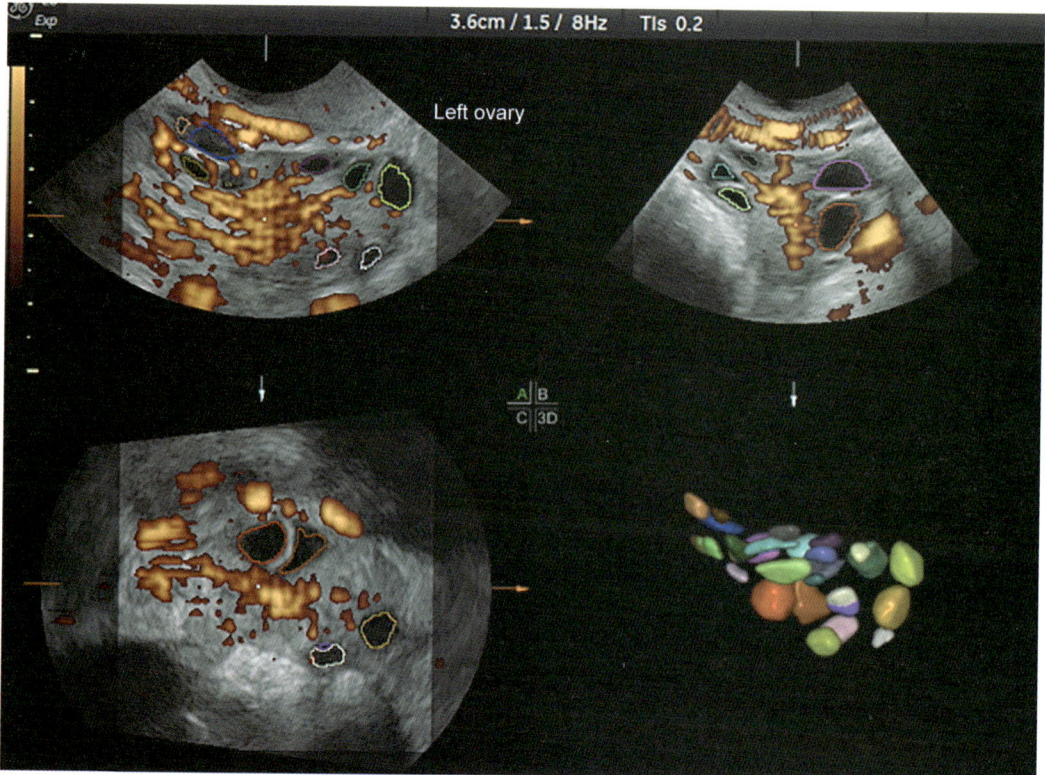

Fig. 1: 3D ultrasound image of the ovary with SonoAVC for calculating antral follicle counts. (SonoAVC: sonography-based automated volume count)

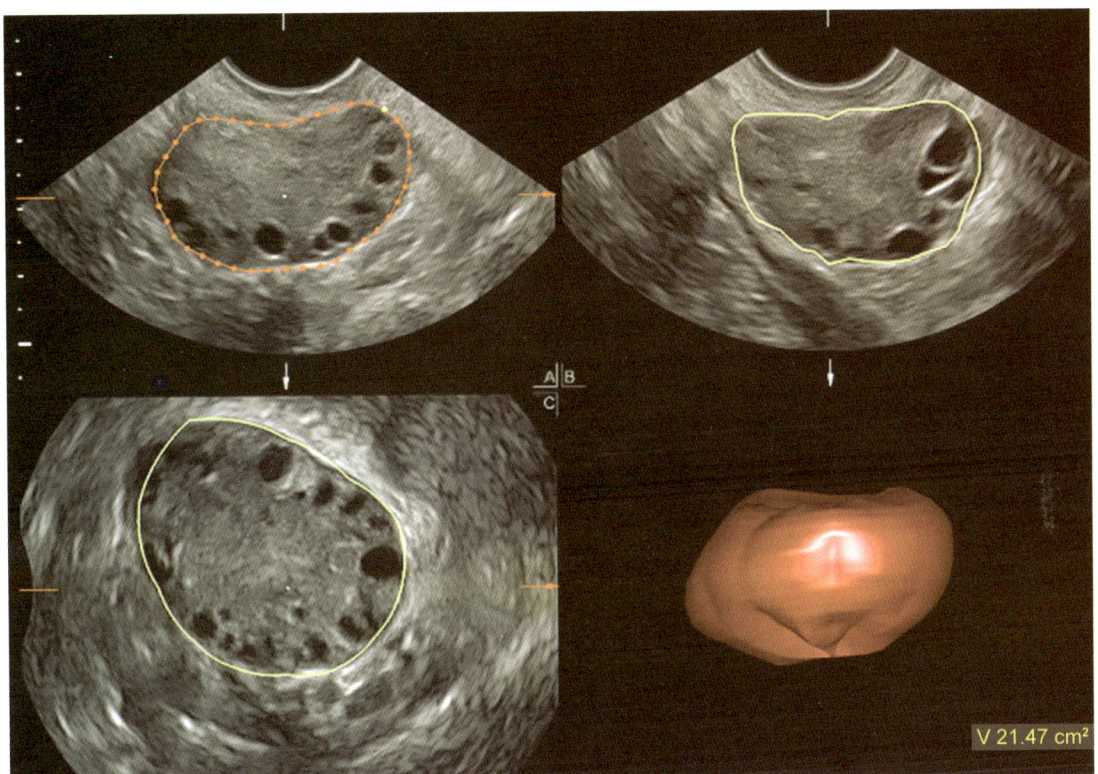

Fig. 2: 3D ultrasound calculated ovarian volume by a software called VOCAL. (VOCAL: virtual organ computer-aided analysis)

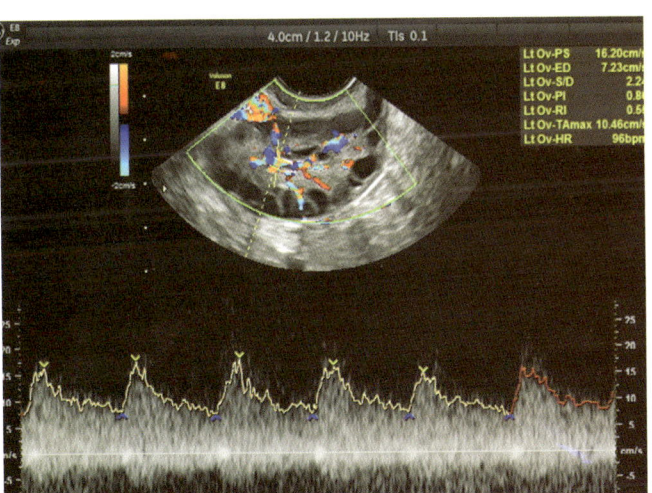

Fig. 3: Ovarian stromal flow as seen on color Doppler and pulse Doppler.

across the ovary in longitudinal and transverse axes to find large vessels seen in their long axis, and these can be traced outside the ovarian margins also. These are ovarian artery and ovarian branch of uterine artery. The plane in which these vessels are seen is the hilar plane. Scroll the probe across on both sides from this plane and find the brightest vessels in the stroma, away from the hilar plane and away from the follicles. These are stromal vessels. Measure the flow with a pulsed wave Doppler with sample volume of 2 mm.

The total number of antral follicles and ovarian stromal blood flow were the two most significant predictors of ovarian response and ovarian volume was a highly significant predictor of number of follicles.[3]

Even in old-age patients or patients with endometriosis or patients with polycystic ovarian syndrome, stromal flows are a reliable parameter to decide ovarian response to stimulation.

Consider age and body mass index (BMI) also to calculate the stimulation dose. Age is known to be one of the most important factors that reduces not only the ovarian reserve but also the oocyte quality.

Ultrasound parameters, age, and BMI are reliable parameters for a decision on stimulation doses.[2] AFC is predictive of number of follicles (S. estradiol level) on the day of trigger and BMI was predictive of gonadotropins dosage.[10] Baseline scoring system was developed based on the above mentioned evidences.[11,12]

Baseline scoring system is given in **Table 1**.

TABLE 1: Baseline scores depending on the values of age, BMI, AFC, ovarian volume, stromal RI, and stromal PSV.

Score	1	2	3	4	5
Age	>40	35.1–40	30.1–35	25.1–30	<25
BMI	>30	30–28.1	28–25.1	25–22.1	<22
AFC	<5	5–10	10–15	15–20	>20
Ovarian volume	<3	3.1–5	5.1–7	7.1–10	>10
Stromal RI	>0.75	0.75–0.66	0.65–0.56	0.55–0.45	<0.45
Stromal PSV	<3	3.1–5	5.1–7	7.1–10	>10

(AFC: antral follicle count; BMI: body mass index; PSV: peak systolic velocity; RI: resistance index)

Depending on the baseline score, the doses of recombinant follicle-stimulating hormone (rFSH) for ovulation induction are as follows **(Table 2)**:

*For IUI cycles **(Flowchart 2)**:*
Transvaginal scan is done to assess the size of the follicles on the day when the gonadotropins are to be started. If follicle is already larger than 10 mm and also shows some perifollicular flow (vessels overlapping on the follicular wall), it is a dominant follicle. In this case, the follicle has already become FSH sensitive, will respond to FSH, and will grow at a rate of approximately 2 mm a day. Calculate when it is likely to reach 17–18 mm and accordingly call the patient. If all the follicles are smaller than 10 mm, the patient is directly called after 5 days of gonadotropin stimulation.

If on day 5, the follicle and endometrium both have not grown, then it is considered nonresponse and in these cases, dose of gonadotropin needs to be modified as mentioned below in IUI cycles depending on what was the baseline score.

It is important to remember here that for IUI cycles done with only oral ovulogens, baseline scoring is not required.

*For IVF cycles **(Flowchart 3)**:*
As per the results of our study,[11,12] the scoring system devised in this study for deciding the gonadotropin dose is highly reliable for safe planning of stimulation protocols in IUI cycles as the ovarian hyperstimulation syndrome (OHSS) rates and cycle cancellation rates due to poor response are negligible. The conception rate is also decent, 35–40% per IUI cycle. Even in polycystic ovary syndrome (PCOS) patients, it conveniently gives the most bi/tri follicular development. Multiple pregnancy rates are also acceptable.

The parameters for IUI and IVF are given in **Table 3**.

TABLE 2: Doses of rFSH to be given for ovulation induction in patients undergoing IUI, IVF fresh transfer, or IVF frozen transfer cycles.

Score	IUI	IVF	IVF FET
≥25	25 IU	75 IU	150 IU
21–25	37.5 IU	150 IU	225 IU
16–20	75 IU	225 IU	300 IU
11–15	112.5 IU	300 IU	375 IU
6–10	150 IU	375 IU	450 IU

(FET: frozen embryo transfer; IUI: intrauterine insemination; IVF: in vitro fertilization; rFSH: recombinant follicle-stimulating hormone)

Flowchart 2: Algorithm to be followed for the intrauterine insemination (IUI) cycle in case of no response on day 5 of ovulation induction.

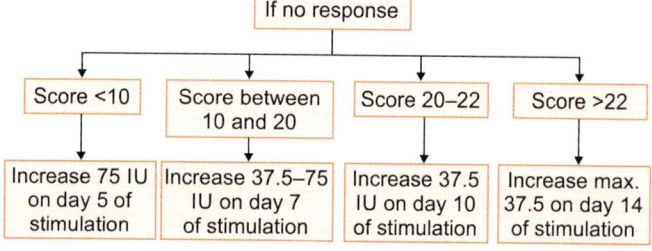

Flowchart 3: Algorithm to be followed for in vitro fertilization (IVF) cycle in case of no response on day 5 of ovulation induction.

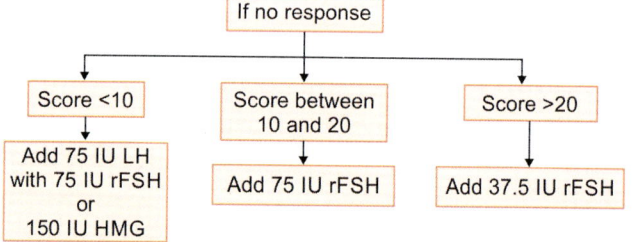

(HMG: human menopausal gonadotropins; LH: luteinizing hormone; rFSH: recombinant follicle-stimulating hormone)

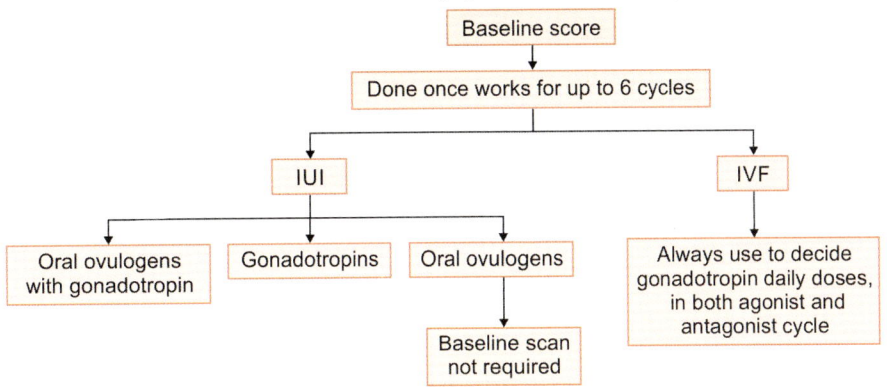

Flowchart 4: Baseline scoring system in IUI and IVF cycles.

(IUI: intrauterine insemination; IVF: in vitro fertilization)

TABLE 3: Parameters selection for IUI and IVF.

Parameter	IUI	IVF
Age	As it is	As it is
BMI	As it is	As it is
AFC	Total of both ovaries	Total of both ovaries
Ovarian volume	One with the better flow	Mean
Stromal RI	Of the ovary with lower RI	Mean
Stromal PSV	Of the ovary with lower RI	Mean

(AFC: antral follicle count; BMI: body mass index; IUI: intrauterine insemination; IVF: in vitro fertilization; PSV: peak systolic velocity; RI: resistance index)

REFERENCES

1. Krishnakumar J, Agarwal A, Nambiar D, Radhakrishnan S. Comparison of antral follicle count, antimullerian hormone and day 2 follicle stimulating hormone as predictor of ovarian response and clinical pregnancy rate in patient with an abnormal ovarian reserve test. Int J Reprod Contracept Obstet Gynecol. 2016;5(8):2762-7.
2. Freiesleben NL, Lossl K, Bogstad J, Bredkjaer HE, Toft B, Loft A, et al. Predictors of ovarian response in intrauterine insemination patients and development of a dosage nomogram. Reprod Biomed Online. 2008;17(5):632-41.
3. Popovic-Todorovic B, Loft A, Lindhard A, Bangsbøll S, Andersson AM, Andersen AN. A prospective study of predictive factors of ovarian response in 'standard' IVF/ICSI patients treated with recombinant FSH. A suggestion for recombinant FSH dosage normogram. Hum Reprod. 2003;18(4):781-7.
4. Lass A, Skull J, McVeigh E, Margara R, Winston RM. Measurement of ovarian volume by transvaginal sonography before ovulation induction with human menopausal gonadotrophin for in vitro fertilization can predict poor response. Hum Reprod. 1997;12(2):294-7.
5. Mercé LT, Barco MJ, Bau S, Troyano JM. Prediction of ovarian response and IVF/ICSI outcome by three dimensional ultrasonography and power Doppler angiography. Eur J Obstet Gynecol Reprod Biol. 2007;132(1):93-100.
6. te Velde ER. Advances in fertility studies and reproductive medicine [thesis]. Durban: International Federation of Fertility Societies; 2007. p. 306.
7. Zaidi J, Barber J, Kyei-Mensah A, Bekir J, Campbell S, Tan SL. Relationship of ovarian stromal blood flow at baseline ultrasound to subsequent follicular response in an in vitro fertilization program. Obstet Gynecol. 1996;88(5):779-84.
8. Engmann L, Saldkevicius P, Agrawal R, Bekir JS, Campbell S, Tan SL. Value of ovarian stromal blood flow velocity measurement after pituitary suppression in the prediction of ovarian responsiveness and outcome of in vitro fertilization treatment. Fertil Steril. 1999;71(1):22-9.
9. Arora A, Gainder S, Dhaliwal L, Suri V. Clinical significance of ovarian stromal blood flow in assessment of ovarian response in stimulated cycle for in vitro fertilization. Int J Reprod Contracept Obstet Gynecol. 2015;4(5):1380-3.
10. Ng EH, Tang OS, Chan CC, Ho PC. Ovarian stromal blood flow in the prediction of ovarian response during in vitro fertilization treatment. Hum Reprod. 2005;20(11):3147-51.
11. Panchal S, Nagori C. Ultrasound-based decision making on stimulation protocol for superovulated intrauterine insemination cycles. Int J Infertil Fetal Med. 2016;7(1):7-13.
12. Panchal S, Nagori C. Ultrasound Based decision making on stimulation protocol in IVF. Donald School J Ultrasound Obstet Gynecol. 2016;10(3):330-7.

Preovulatory Assessment

INTRODUCTION

Ultrasound (US) and hormonal assessment are considered two primary investigations for evaluation of female factor of infertility. With advancing US technology, Doppler and 3D US have eliminated the need for majority of other investigations for cycle monitoring. When US is used with Doppler, it gives precise idea about not only the morphological changes but also vascular changes occurring during the entire cycle. Vascular changes are instantaneous to hormonal changes and occur before morphological changes.

WHEN IS THE FOLLICLE FUNCTIONALLY MATURE?

Follicle gains dominance at a mean diameter of approximately 10 mm and it grows at a rate of 2–3 mm per day. As the dominant follicle grows, it starts pulling vascularity toward itself.[1,2] This is to allow the exposure of the follicle to follicle-stimulating hormone (FSH) and development of FSH receptors on the follicle.

Follicle, that grows to >16–17 mm **(Fig. 1)** in diameter [follicular diameter is measured as single anteroposterior (AP) diameter, when the follicle is seen as a spherical structure or three longest orthogonal diameters must be measured in two orthogonal planes and the mean is used as follicular diameter] has anechoic contents, thin isoechoic wall, is round or oval, and grows at a rate of 2–3 mm/day could be considered a mature follicle on 2D US alone. A thin hypoechoic rim can be seen surrounding the follicle 24–36 hours before ovulation. Cumulus-like shadow may be seen at same time (in about 35–40% of mature follicles—not a mandatory sign for follicle maturity evaluation).

Low-level echogenicities are seen inside the follicle parallel to the wall about 6–10 hours before rupture, due to separation of the inner wall **(Fig. 2)**. Around the same time, irregularity of the follicle wall is seen due to triangular anechoic niche-like shadows. And both these later signs are considered to be signs of impending ovulation.

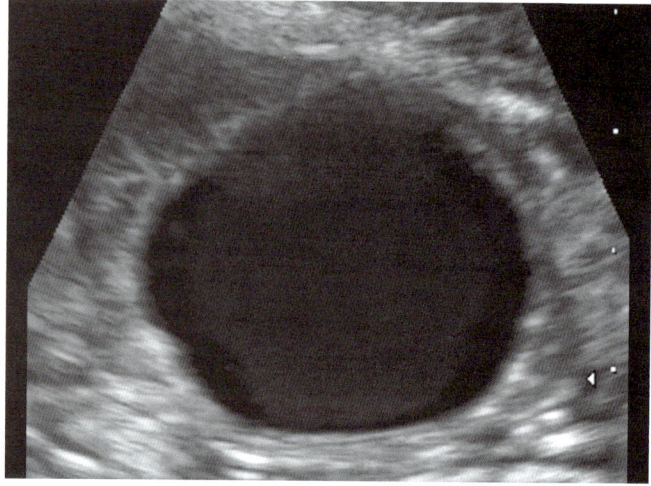

Fig. 1: B-mode ultrasound image of a mature follicle.

On Doppler:

The blood vessels that have started growing toward the dominant follicle gradually increase to cover 2/3–3/4 of follicular circumference **(Fig. 3)**. Fall in perifollicular resistance index (RI) starts 2 days before ovulation.[3] These vessels show RI of 0.4–0.48[4] and this correlates with the preovulatory estrogen surge. It speaks about the adequacy of estrogen production by the follicle and thus about follicle quality. Then peak systolic velocity (PSV) starts rising and when PSV reaches 10 cm/sec, it is the time for the natural surge or the time to give surrogate surge in case a patient is under fertility treatment **(Fig. 4)**. Preovulatory perifollicular PSV correlates with the luteinizing hormone (LH) levels.

But when assessing perifollicular flows, ovarian stromal flows, corpus luteal flows, and endometrial flows,

Preovulatory Assessment

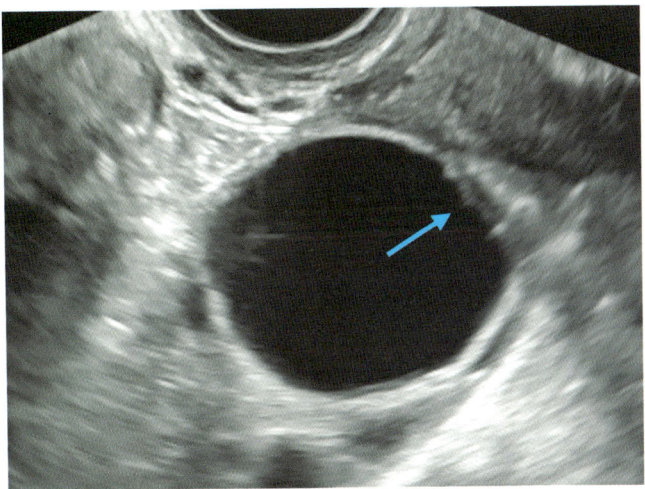

Fig. 2: B-mode ultrasound image of a follicle of which rupture is impending showing mild separation of inner wall (blue arrow) at 2 o'clock and 6 o'clock positions.

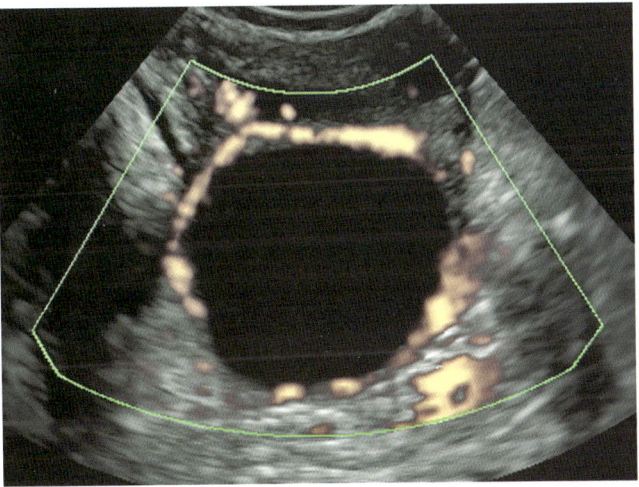

Fig. 3: Perifollicular vascularity seen on color Doppler.

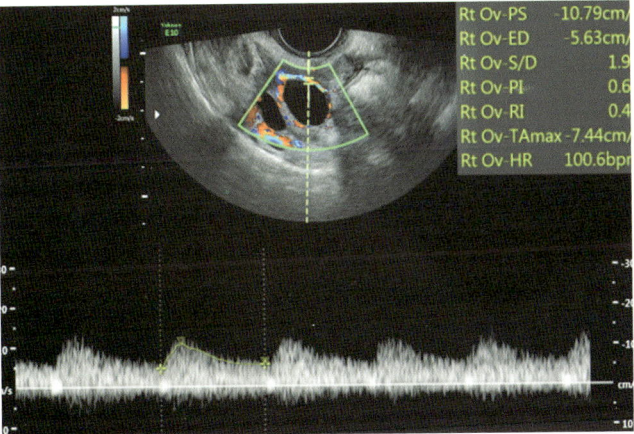

Fig. 4: Pulse Doppler image of the low resistance perifollicular flow.

remember that the pulse repetition frequency (PRF) is always set at 0.3 for color and power Doppler, with wall motion filter at the latest and gains once set in the preset should not be changed. Also, remember that the vessels that overlap on the follicular wall are perifollicular vessels. Flow may be assessed on the brightest color spots. RI and PSV matching only in one vessel with 2/3 to 3/4 circumference of the follicle covered by blood vessels is sufficient to confirm follicle maturity.

Why is Doppler assessment essential?

- Ovarian flow correlates well with oocyte recovery rates.
- Embryos produced by fertilization of the ova obtained from the follicles that had a perifollicular PSV of <10 cm/sec are less likely to be grade I embryos and also have higher chance of chromosomal malformations.[5,6]
- Oocytes from severely hypoxic follicles are associated with high frequency of abnormalities of organization of chromosomes on metaphase spindle and may lead to segregation disorders and catastrophic mosaics in embryo.[7]

On 3D ultrasound:

Follicular volume of 3–7.5 cm^3, calculated by virtual organ computer-aided analysis (VOCAL) software of 3D US has been found to be optimum in our study.[8] This agrees with the study by Wittmaack et al,[9] which says that in in vitro fertilization–embryo transfer (IVF-ET) cycles, follicles with mean follicular diameter of 12–24 mm are associated with optimal rates of oocyte recovery, fertilization, and cleavage.[9] This corresponds to the follicular volumes of between 3.77 and 7.54 mL **(Fig. 5)**. Volume assessment of the follicles is especially important when there is multifollicular development and the follicles are compressed by each other leading to irregular shape. In such a situation, mean diameter of three longest orthogonal diameters is not precise and neither the VOCAL nor the sonography-based automated volume count (SonoAVC) software of 3D US.

Follicles containing oocytes capable to produce a pregnancy have a perifollicular vascular network more uniform and distinctive.[10] In our study,[8] perifollicular vascularization index (VI) of 6–20 and perifollicular flow index (FI) >35 are most optimum. 3D power Doppler gives the most precise information about the vascularization and follicular blood flow.[11]

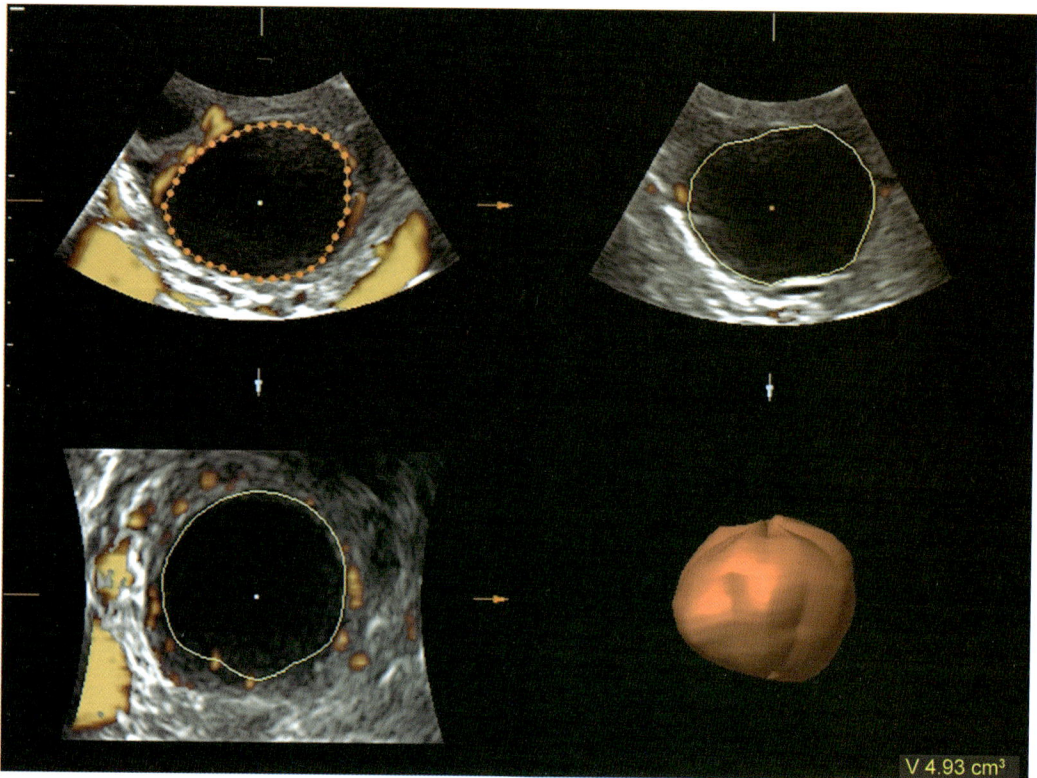

Fig. 5: 3D ultrasound acquired, virtual organ computer-aided analysis (VOCAL) calculated volume of follicle.

After surge starts:
When perifollicular PSV is 10 cm/sec, it is the time when the LH surge starts and under the effect of that LH, the perifollicular PSV keeps on rising constantly.[12] Vascular changes at the time of impending ovulation include increased vascularity of the inner wall of the follicle and a coincident surge in blood velocity just prior to eruption.[12] This derives that a rising PSV with steady low RI suggests that the follicle is close to rupture. Therefore, in cases where on pretrigger scan, the follicular PSV is high with low RI, it is an indication of the start of the surge, which means ovulation starting earlier than 36–42 hours and in these cases, earlier intrauterine insemination (IUI) gives better results. One may also plan double IUI, one at 12–14 hours and another at 36–38 hours after trigger. This covers the entire period of likely ovulation and the results of IUI are better.

WHAT INDICATES GOOD ENDOMETRIAL RECEPTIVITY?

B-mode features of endometrium with good receptivity:
- Minimum endometrial thickness of 6 mm but 8–10 mm is optimum. The endometrial morphology may be grade A, B, or C. Grade A, when it is a triple line

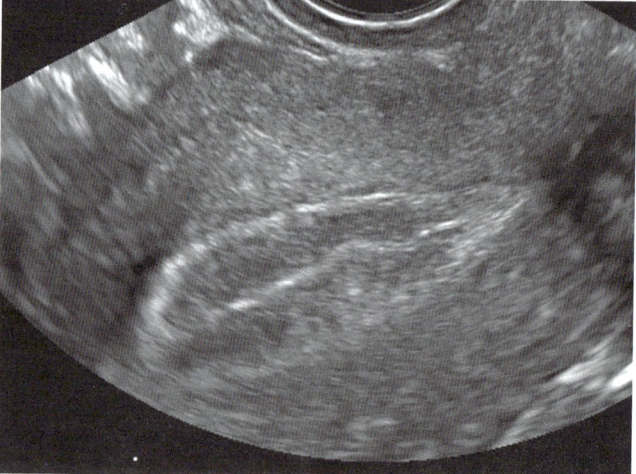

Fig. 6: B-mode ultrasound image of grade-A endometrium.

endometrium with the intervening area as echogenic as the anterior myometrium and usually relates with 3–5 mature follicles **(Fig. 6)**. Grade B **(Fig. 7),** when it is multilayered or triple line with hypoechoic intervening area and relates with 1–2 mature follicles. Grade C, when it is homogeneous isoechoic endometrium[13] and represents **(Fig. 8)**. It is important to remember

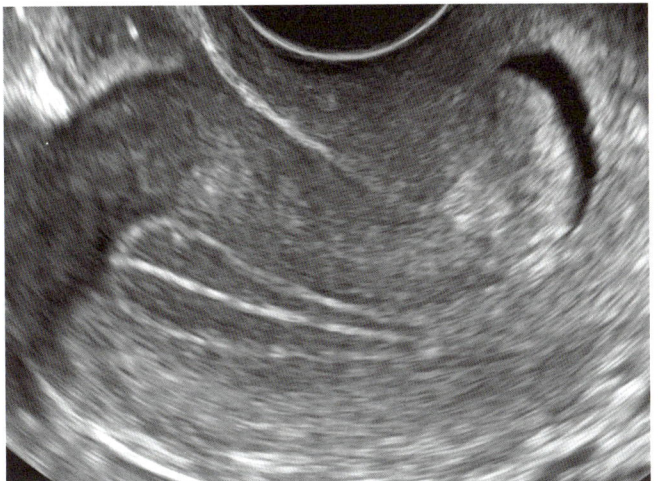

Fig. 7: B-mode ultrasound image of grade-B endometrium.

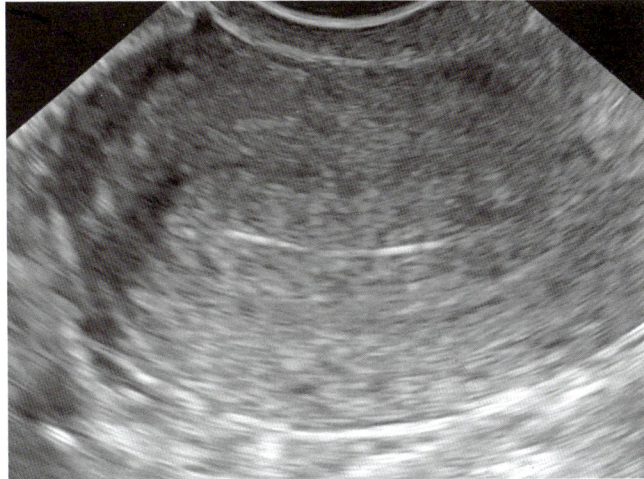

Fig. 8: B-mode ultrasound image of grade-C endometrium.

here that even grade C is a pure estrogen-dominated endometrium and relates with multifollicular development, and the changes in morphology indicate the amount of estrogen.

Doppler features of endometrium with good receptivity:
Implantation rates correlate more to the vascularity of the endometrium rather than the thickness and morphology of the endometrium.

On Doppler, endometrium shows vascularity in zones 3 and 4 or maybe called subendometrial and endometrial layers **(Figs. 9A to D)**.

The zones of vascularity are defined according to Applebaum[14] as zone 1, when the vascularity on power Doppler is seen only at endometriomyometrium junction; zone 2, when vessels penetrate through the hyperechogenic endometrial edge; zone 3, when it reaches intervening hypoechogenic zone; and zone 4, when they reach the endometrial cavity and only covers at least 5 mm^2 area of that zone.

Absent flow in the endometrial and subendometrial zones on the day of trigger indicates total failure of implantation.[15]

These arteries should have an RI <0.6. On pulse Doppler of the uterine artery, pulsatility index (PI) should be <3.2 **(Fig. 10)**.[16,17]

Endometrial Vascularity: Its Relation to Implantation Rates (Nagori and Panchal)[18]

Endometrial vascularity is given in **Table 1**.

On 3D ultrasound:
Endometrial volume assessment by 3D US volume calculation correlates the cycle outcome with quantitative parameter rather than endometrial thickness.[9] This is done by a software called VOCAL. Pregnancy and implantation rates were significantly lower when endometrial volume was <2 mL.[19,20]

To summarize **(Table 2)**:
If these parameters are not reached, the cycle is not canceled, only trigger is delayed. Stimulation is continued till these parameters are achieved. In case if the PSV of the follicle starts rising with low RI, it means the ovulation is impending. In such a situation, in spite of inadequate endometrial parameters, the trigger is given, but the patient is also explained that the result cannot be as good as it would be if every parameter was optimal. If the follicle grows beyond 23–24 mm and still perifollicular flow is not adequate, trigger is planned and patient may be given a choice of either timed intercourse or IUI, after proper explanation about the results.

After the surge has started:
The PSV of the perifollicular vessels increases, and higher PSV indicates advanced surge and ovulation earlier than 36–42 hours. In such cases, it is an IUI cycle; IUI needs to be planned earlier than 36–38 hours to achieve the best possible conception rate.

With the advancing LH surge, estrogen level falls leading to decrease in endometrial thickness by 0.5 mm and there is also decrease in endometrial vascularity. Progesterone normally also rises before ovulation, after

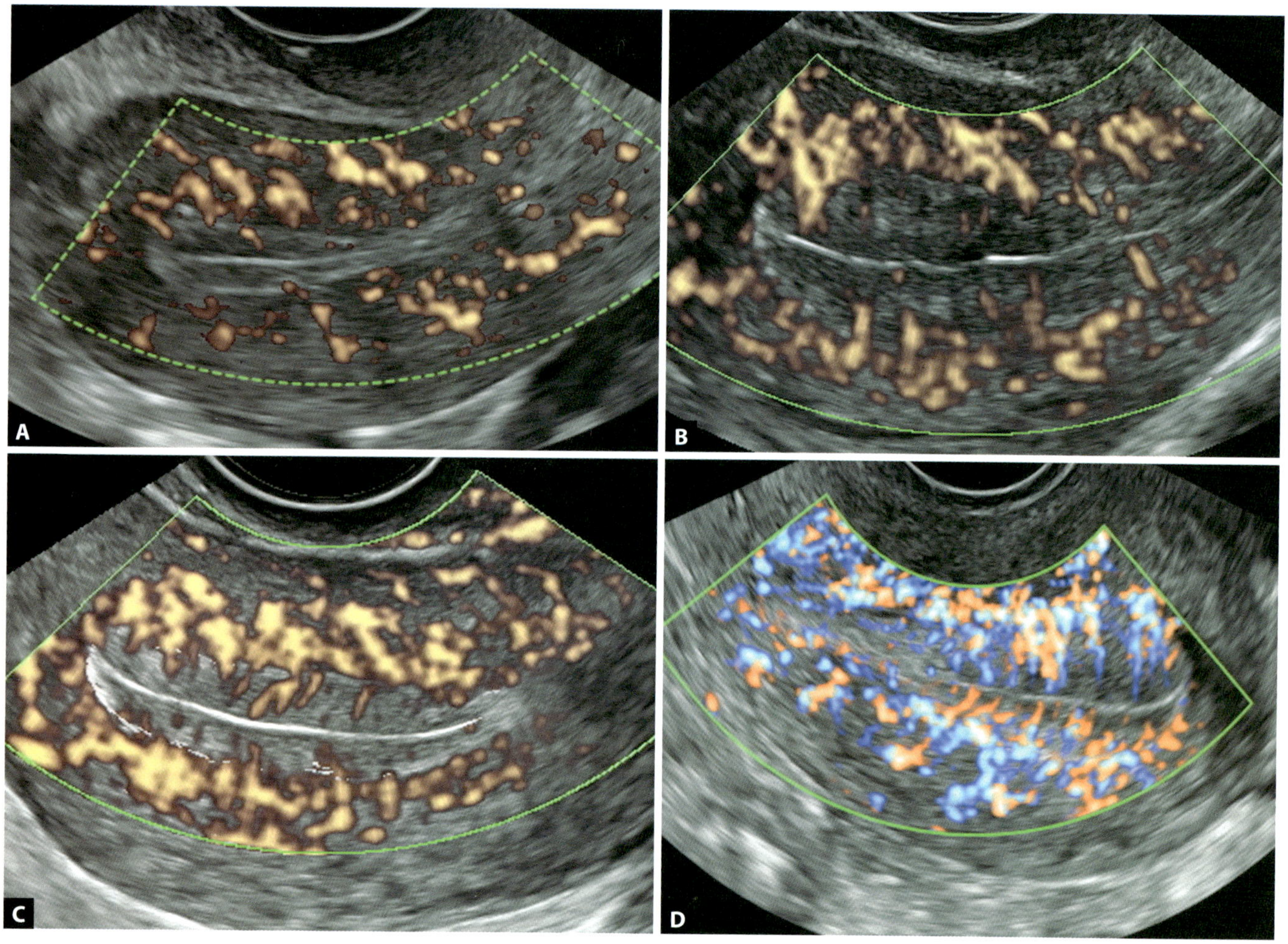

Figs. 9A to D: Power Doppler images of the grade 1–4 endometrium.

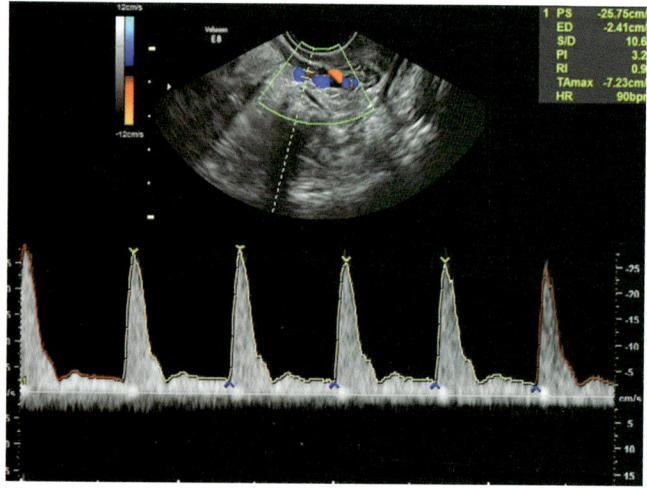

Fig. 10: Pulse Doppler image showing high resistance uterine artery flow waveform.

TABLE 1: Endometrial vascularity.				
Vascularity in	Zone 1	Zone 2	Zone 3	Zone 4
% of patients	6.69%	20.73%	58%	14.47%
+ βhCG	19%	21.87%	39.77%	70.14
Gestational sac	9.6%	14.58%	36.8%	68.65%
Abortions	50%	23.8%	5.6%	1.5%
(hCG: human chorionic gonadotropin)				

the surge starts. This shows fluffiness of outer margin of multilayered endometrium **(Fig 11)**. This indicates physiological level of progesterone and exposure duration of up to 24 hours. It also indicates good endometrial receptivity. With this, there is also rise in uterine artery PI on the dominant side.

When the progesterone level rises beyond the physiological levels or exposure of progesterone to

TABLE 2: Preovulatory follicle and endometrium.		
	Follicle	**Endometrium**
Size/thickness	16–18 mm	8–10 mm
Morphology	Thin wall, no internal echoes, halo	Grade A/B
Vascularity	3/4th circumference	Zone 3–4
Resistance index	0.4–0.48	<0.5
Peak systolic velocity	>10 cm/sec	–
Uterine artery pulsatility index	–	<3.2
Volume	3–7 cm^3	3–7 cm^3
3D morphology	Cumulus	Intact endometriomyometrium junction
3D Power Doppler	More symmetrical the better	Higher the better

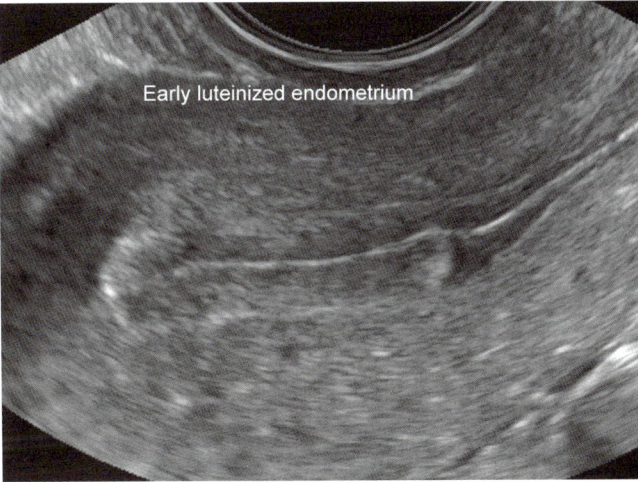

Fig. 11: Endometrium of early luteal phase seen on B-mode ultrasound. It shows fluffiness of outer margins of multilayered endometrium.

endometrium is too long, and starts deteriorating the endometrial receptivity, the outer margin of endometrium starts becoming hyperechoic.

These changes in the endometrium with immature follicle indicate premature LH surge whereas with rupture of the follicle indicates recent ovulation.

Preovulatory scan:
- Confirm dominance of the follicle by perifollicular blood flow and not by 10 mm size.
- *Good quality follicle (2D):* Anechoic, thin isoechoic wall, round/oval shape, and growth rate of 2–3 mm a day

- *Pretrigger follicle:* Apart from above-mentioned criteria
- *On 2D:* Mean follicular diameter of 16–18 mm at least
  - Hypoechoic halo starts appearing before 24–36 hours of ovulation.
  - Cumulus-like shadow starts appearing before 24–36 hours of ovulation.
  - *Low-level internal echogenicities in follicle lumen, parallel to follicular wall:* 6–12 hours before ovulation
  - *Rosebush thorn sign:* 5–10 hours before ovulation
- *On color Doppler (CD):* Vascularity covering at least 2/3 preferable 3/4 of the circumference
  - Perifollicular RI <0.48
  - Perifollicular PSV >10 cm/sec
- *On 3D:* Follicular volume of 3–7cm^3 correlates with diameter of 18–24 mm.
  - SonoAVC gives precise count and size of these follicles.
  - 3D power Doppler gives better idea about global vascularity of the follicle.
  - Cumulus may be visualized in more percentage of mature follicles.
- **Good quality endometrium**
- *On 2D ultrasound:*
  - Thickness at least 6 mm, preferable 8–10 mm
  - Grade A, B, or C
- *On CD:* Intraendometrial flow
  - 5 mm^2 area vascularized
  - Spiral RI <0.6
  - Uterine PI <3.2
- *On 3D:* Endometrial volume at least 2 cc
  - Endometrial global vascularity

CONCLUSION

Ultrasound is an excellent tool to decide the time of trigger and time of IUI. Doppler adds to the information available and for the final fine-tuning of the treatment cycle.

REFERENCES

1. Zaidi J, Barber J, Kyei-Mensah A, Bekir J, Campbell S, Tan SL. Relationship of ovarian stromal blood flow at the baseline ultrasound scan to subsequent follicular response in an in vitro fertilization program. Obstet Gynecol. 1996;88:779-84.
2. Engmann L, Sladkevicius P, Agrawal R, Bekir JS, Campbell S, Tan SL. Value of ovarian stromal blood flow velocity measurement after pituitary suppression in the prediction of ovarian responsiveness and outcome of in vitro fertilization treatment. Fertil Steril. 1999;71(1):22-9.

3. Jokubkeine L, Sladkevicius P, Rovas L, Valentine L. Assessment of changes in volume and vascularity of ovaries during the normal menstrual cycle using three-dimensional power Doppler ultrasound. Hum Reprod. 2006;21(10):2661-8.
4. Kurjak A, Kupesic-Urek S. Infertility. In: Kurjak A (Ed). Transvaginal Color Doppler. Carnforth, UK: Parthenon Publishing; 1991. pp. 33-8.
5. Nargund G, Doyle PE, Bourne TH, Parsons JH, Cheng WC, Campbell S, et al. Ultrasound-derived indices of follicular blood flow before HCG administration and prediction of oocyte recovery and preimplantation embryo quality. Hum Reprod. 1996;11(11):2512-7.
6. Nargund G, Bourne TH, Doyle P, Parsons J, Cheng W, Campbell S, et al. Association between ultrasound indices of follicular blood flow, oocyte recovery and preimplantation embryo quality. Hum Reprod. 1996;11(1):109-13.
7. Van Blerkom J, Antezak M, Schrader R. The developmental potential of human oocyte is related to the dissolved oxygen content of follicular fluid: Association with vascular endothelial growth factor levels and perifollicular blood flow characteristics. Hum Reprod. 1997;12(5):1047-55.
8. Panchal SY, Nagori CB. Can 3D PD be a better tool for assessing the pre-HCG follicle and endometrium? A randomized study of 500 cases. Presented at 16th World Congress on Ultrasound in Obstetrics and Gynecology, 2006, London. J Ultrasound Obstet Gynecol. Sept. 2006; 28(4):504.
9. Wittmaack FM, Kreger DO, Blasco L, Tureck RW, Mastroianni L Jr Lessey BA. Effect of follicular size on oocyte retrieval, fertilization, cleavage and embryo quality in in vitro fertilization cycles: A 6-year data collection. Fertil Steril. 1994;62(6):1205-10.
10. Vlaisavljević V, Reljic M, Gavrić Lovrec V, Zazula D, Sergent N. Measurement of perifollicular blood flow of the dominant preovulatory follicle using three-dimensional power doppler. Ultrasound Obstet Gynecol. 2003;22(5):520-6.
11. Mercé LT, Barco MJ, Kupesic S, Kurjak A. 2D and 3D power doppler ultrasound: From ovulation to implantation. In: Kurjak A, Chervenak F (Eds). Textbook of Perinatal Medicine. London: Parthenon Publishing; 2005.
12. Bourne TH, Jurkovic D, Waterstone J, Campbell S, Collins WP. Intrafollicular blood flow during human ovulation. Ultrasound Obstet Gynecol. 1991;1(1):53-9.
13. Smith B, Porter R, Ahuja K, Craft I. Ultrasonic assessment of endometrial changes in stimulated cycles in an in vitro fertilization and embryo transfer program. J In Vitro Fert Embryo Transf. 1984;1:233-8.
14. Applebaum M. The 'steel' or 'teflon' endometrium-ultrasound visualization of endometrial vascularity in IVF patients and outcome. Presented at the third World Congress of Ultrasound in Obstetrics and Gynecology. Ultrasound Obstet Gynecol 1993;3(Suppl 2):10.
15. Zaidi J, Campbell S, Pittrof R, Tan SL. Endometrial thickness, morphology, vascular penetration and velocimetry in predicting implantation in an in vitro fertilization program. Ultrasound Obstet Gynecol. 1995;6(3):191-8.
16. Steer CV, Campbell S, Tan SL, Crayford T, Mills C, Mason BA, et al. The use of transvaginal color flow imaging after in vitro fertilization to identify optimum uterine conditions before embryo transfer. Fertil Steril. 1992;57(2):372-6.
17. Zaidi J, Pittrof R, Shaker A, Kyei-Mensah A, Campbell S, Tan SL. Assessment of uterine artery blood flow on the day of human chorionic gonadotrophin administration by transvaginal color Doppler ultrasound in an in vitro fertilization program. Fertil Steril. 1996;65(2):377-81.
18. Nagori C, Panchal S. Endometrial vascularity: Its relation to implantation rates IJIFM. 2012;3(2):48-50
19. Raga F, Bonilla-Musoles F, Casañ EM, Klein O, Bonilla F. Assessment of endometrial volume by three-dimensional ultrasound prior to embryo transfer: Clues to endometrial receptivity. Hum Reprod. 1999;14(11):2851-4.
20. Kupesic S, Bekavac I, Bjelos D, Kurjak A. Assessment of endometrial receptivity by transvaginal color Doppler and three-dimensional power doppler ultrasonography in patients undergoing in vitro fertilization procedures. J Ultrasound Med. 2001;20:125-34.

Luteal Phase Scan

Chapter 22

Rupture of the follicle leads to formation of corpus luteum and initiation of the luteal phase of the cycle. Corpus luteum is responsible for progesterone production. But the level of progesterone is very low in early proliferative phase and it is only during midproliferative phase that progesterone level reaches a plateau. Therefore, assessment of the luteal phase must always be done in the midluteal phase. The functional efficacy of the corpus luteum can be assessed by Doppler by assessing the pericorpus luteal vascularity.

Segmental uterine and ovarian artery perfusion demonstrates a significant correlation with histological and hormonal markers of uterine receptivity and may aid the assessment of luteal phase defect.[1] A clear correlation between resistance index (RI) of corpus luteum and plasma progesterone levels has been seen in a natural cycle. RI of the corpus luteum can therefore be used as an adjunct to plasma progesterone assay as an index of luteal function.[2]

A corpus luteum that is functionally normal and produces an adequate amount of progesterone shows corpus luteal flow: RI = 0.35 – 0.50 and peak systolic velocity (PSV) = 10 – 15 cm/sec **(Figs. 1A and B)**.

The receptor organ for progesterone also (like estrogen) is endometrium and its vascular studies can be a reliable clue to adequate progesterone production. Endometrium also becomes hyperechoic as a result of progesterone exposure and increases in thickness. Normal endometrial thickness is 2 mm more than the preovulatory thickness. But soon after the rupture of the follicle, the outer margin of the endometrium starts becoming fluffy and blurred. With adequate progesterone levels, that are achieved in the midluteal phase, the spiral arteries show RI of 0.48–0.52 (low resistance flow) and uterine artery shows pulsatility index (PI) of 2.0–2.5 **(Figs. 2A and B)**. This PI is lower than in the preovulatory phase because of smooth-muscle relaxing effect of progesterone.

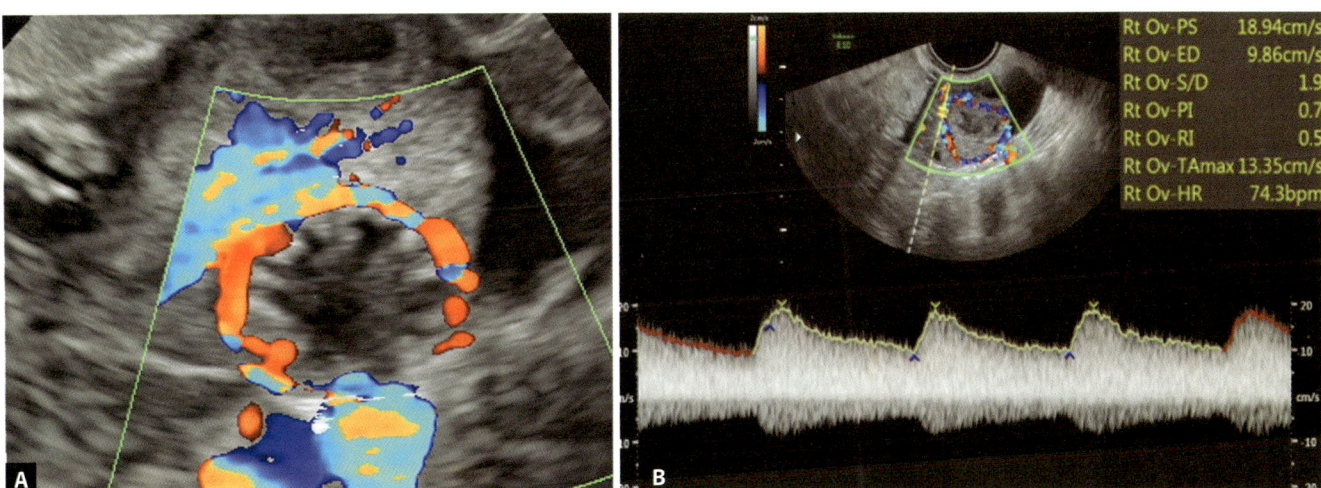

Figs. 1A and B: Normal corpus luteal flow seen on color Doppler and pulse Doppler.

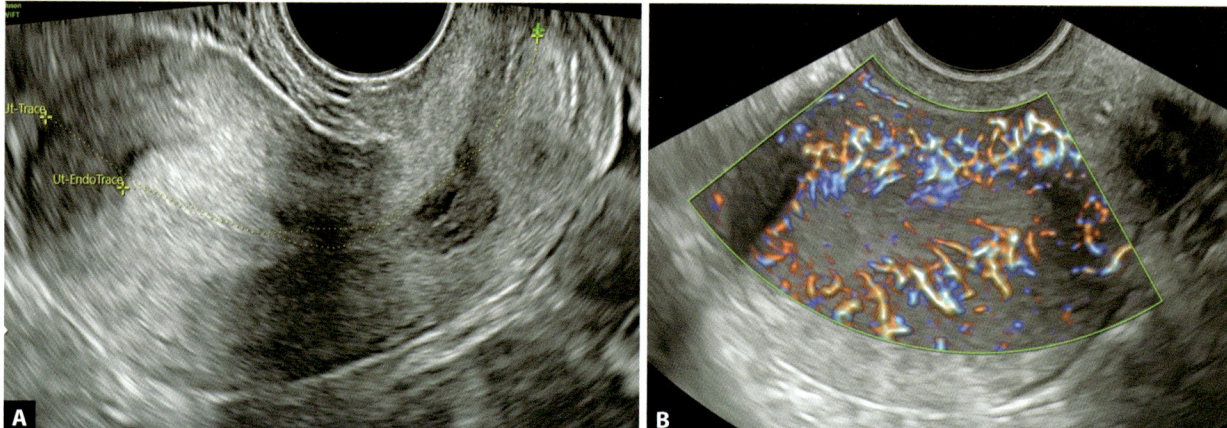

Figs. 2A and B: (A) B-mode ultrasound image of secretory endometrium; (B) HD flow Doppler showing flow in the normal secretory endometrium.

Inadequate progesterone production and, therefore, corpus luteal inadequacy is suggested by high resistance flow in corpus luteal vessels.[2] Whereas high spiral artery resistance would suggest inadequate response of endometrium to progesterone. This is because of inadequate progesterone receptors in the endometrium or because of local endometrial causes, such as endometrial injury or chronic endometritis.

In luteal phase defect because of low progesterone levels, the resistance in the pericorpus luteal vessels is high. Because of low progesterone levels, there is inadequate relaxation of the muscularis of the uterine artery, and therefore the uterine artery resistance is high along with higher resistance in its branches—the spiral vessels.

Corpus luteal flow and spiral artery flow gradient between normal cycle and luteal phase defect:[1] **(Tables 1 and 2)**

Secretory scan is especially helpful in pinpointing the cause of failure of treatment and changing the protocol, if

TABLE 1: Corpus luteal Doppler parameters throughout the cycle in normal cases and in LPD.

	Normal	LPD
Perifollicular	0.56 ± 0.06	0.58 ± 0.04
LH peak day	0.44 ± 0.04	0.58 ± 0.04
Midluteal phase	0.42 ± 0.06	0.58 ± 0.04
Late luteal phase	0.50 ± 0.04	0.58 ± 0.04

(LH: luteinizing hormone; LPD: luteal phase defect)

TABLE 2: Control RI and LPD RI in different phases of a cycle.

Phase	Control RI	LPD RI
Periovulatory	0.53 ± 0.04	0.70 ± 0.06
Mid luteal	0.50 ± 0.02	0.72 ± 0.06
Late luteal	0.51 ± 0.04	0.72 ± 0.04

(LPD: luteal phase defect; RI: resistance index)

Flowchart 1: Algorithm showing diagnosis of normal and abnormal luteal phase.

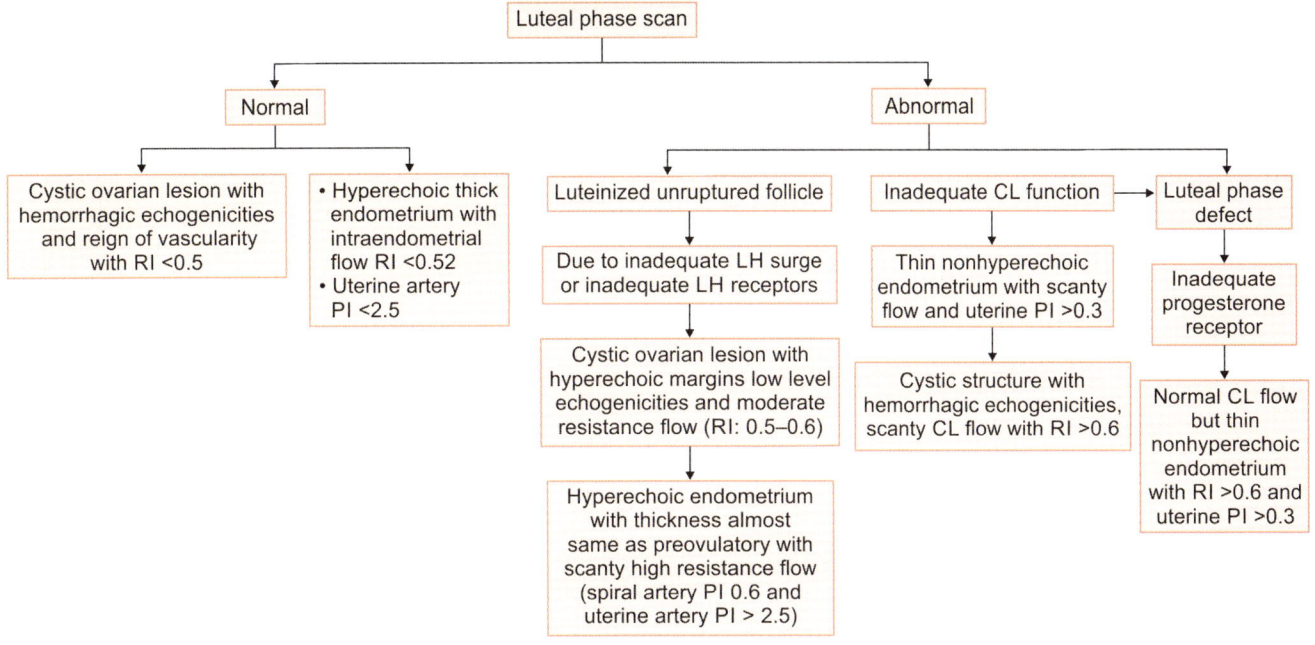

(CL: corpus luteum; LH: luteinizing hormone; PI: pulsatility index; RI: resistance index)

required in the next cycle, for example, human chorionic gonadotropin (hCG) for luteal support in case of corpus luteal failure, more closer monitoring of the cycle and proper time of trigger for luteinized unruptured follicle, and modification in the stimulation protocol for inadequate progesterone receptors in the endometrium.

Diagnosis of normal and abnormal luteal phase is illustrated in **Flowchart 1**.

REFERENCES

1. Kupesić S, Kurjak A, Vujisić S, Petrović Z. Luteal phase defect: comparison between Doppler velocimetry, histological and hormonal markers. Ultrasound Obstet Gynecol. 1997;9(2):105-12.
2. Glock JL, Brumsted JR. Color flow pulsed Doppler ultrasound in diagnosing luteal phase defect. Fertil Steril. 1995;64(3):500-4.

Ultrasound Diagnosis of Polycystic Ovarian Syndrome

POLYCYSTIC OVARIES ON ULTRASOUND

Diagnosis of polycystic ovary syndrome (PCOS) has been a controversial and debatable issue always. Earliest description of polycystic ovaries appears to date from 1845 as "sclerocystic ovaries".[1] Other names suggested are polyfollicular syndrome or ovarian dysmetabolic syndrome. Three major ways for diagnosis of PCOS are: (1) clinical findings, (2) laboratory testing, and (3) ultrasound (US) findings. Approximately, 20–30% of women of reproductive age may have polycystic ovaries, and about half of these have signs and symptoms of PCOS. According to European Society of Human Reproduction and Embryology (ESHRE)/American Society for Reproductive Medicine (ASRM) consensus 2003, the diagnosis of PCOS consists of at least two of the three following criteria:[2]

1. Oligo and/or anovulation
2. *Hyperandrogenism:* Biochemical or clinical
3. *Polycystic ovaries on ultrasound:* This means an ovary that is 10 cm^3 in volume and/or has more than 12 antral follicles.

Though in 2018 and again in 2023, in the ESHRE annual conference, these criteria and the entire Rotterdam consensus for diagnosis of PCOS were revised and according to this revision the follicle number per ovary in PCOS has been changed to 20 per ovary or 10 in the longest section.

Enlarged spherical ovaries more than 10 cm^3 have shown good correlation between ultrasound and diagnosis of polycystic morphology and histopathological criteria for polycystic ovaries.[3] But there are controversies regarding the ovarian enlargement in PCOS.

Since 2003, both a lower threshold of 7 cm and a higher threshold of 13 cm have been proposed as being more appropriate thresholds for polycystic ovarian morphology in different studies.[4,5]

Concerning the ovarian volume (OV), setting the threshold at 7 cm^3 offered the best compromise between specificity (91.2%) and sensitivity (67.5%). In comparison, specificity and sensitivity were 98.2% and 45%, respectively with threshold at 10 cm^3.[6] OV of 6.6 cm^3 has shown 91% sensitivity and 91% specificity for PCOS.[7] Moreover, according to Kupesic, ovaries that are normal in volume can be polycystic as demonstrated by histological and biochemical studies (in 20%). Polycystic ovarian morphology has been found to be a better discriminator than OV between women with PCOS and control women.[8]

Therefore, morphological features of polycystic ovaries need consideration. These include number and arrangement of antral follicles, stromal echogenicity, and vascularity. Though volume of the ovary can be calculated by 2D US by measuring three longest orthogonal diameters or by using 3D software virtual organ computer-aided analysis (VOCAL) **(Figs. 1A and B)**.

ANTRAL FOLLICLE COUNT

Antral follicle count (AFC) is done either by scrolling across the ovary, without rotation and eyeballing, but for PCOS patients, since the number of follicles is plenty, sonography-based automated volume count (SonoAVC)-3D software is more reliable that color codes the follicles and also measures the size of each **(Fig. 2)**.

Antral follicle count of 12 or more (2–9 mm) was used as a characteristic for polycystic ovaries according to Rotterdam criteria (2003), and >20 per ovary according to 2018 amendment in the same. Setting the threshold at 12 for 2–9 mm follicle number per ovary (FNPO) offered the best compromise between specificity (99%) and sensitivity (75%) according to the studies that have been published in 2003–2005.[9] Though polycystic histology and morphology has been found in ovaries having AFC between 5 and 15.

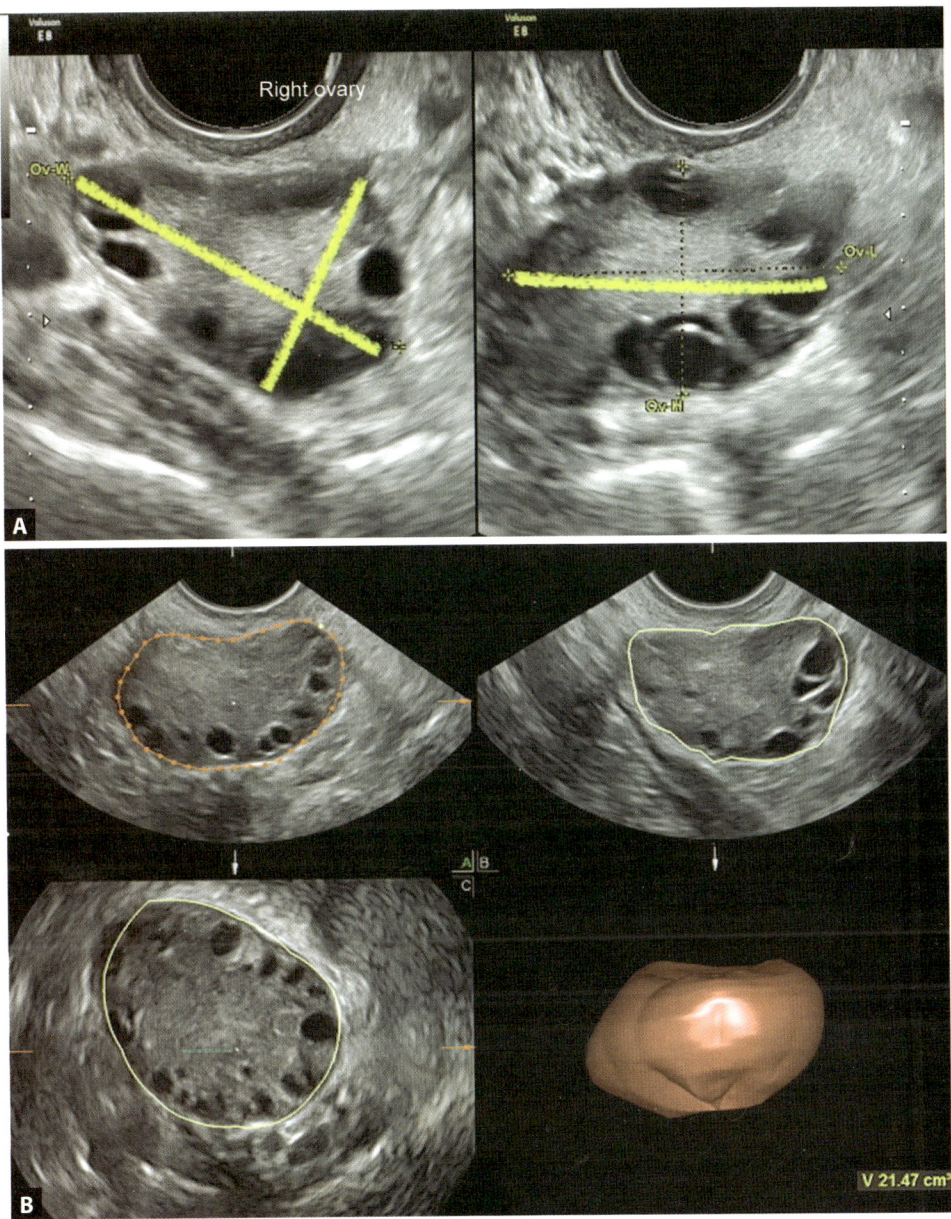

Figs. 1A and B: (A) B-mode ultrasound image of a polycystic ovary with three longest orthogonal diameters taken to calculate the volume; (B) Virtual organ computer-aided analysis (VOCAL) calculated volume of the ovary.

Moreover, it is also known that the AFC is more during the adolescence and decreases as the age advances, so same cutoff cannot be used for different age groups.[10]

European or American population (Caucasian race) with high-frequency transvaginal probes revealed that the diagnostic threshold of the follicle number for PCOS women is about 25.[11-13] Whereas the results of studies conducted by Chen et al. among Chinese women and by Köşüş et al. among Turkish patients indicate lower values (8 and 12, respectively).[14,15] AFC also thus cannot be used as the characteristic of polycystic ovaries.

At this stage a short understanding of pathophysiology and hormonal correlation of ultrasound findings may be helpful.

■ PATHOPHYSIOLOGY

Polycystic ovaries are a result of chronic anovulation. Mildly raised androgen levels, in early follicular phase

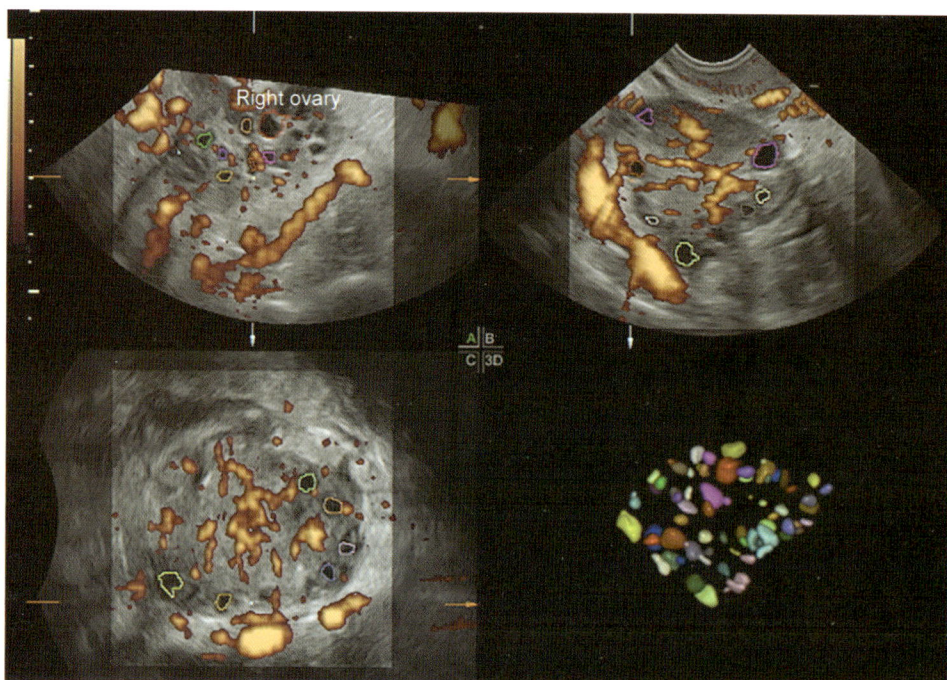

Fig. 2: 3D ultrasound of the polycystic ovary with sonography-based automated volume count (SonoAVC) to calculate the antral follicle count.

in PCOS patients, lead to recruitment of several antral follicles, but further progression does not occur due to hyperinsulinemia and/or other metabolic influences linked to obesity.[9] There is conversion of excess androgen to estrogen and there is also cumulative effect of minimal estradiol production by multiple follicles leading to negative feedback for follicle-stimulating hormone (FSH), and positive feedback for luteinizing hormone (LH). These factors lead to maturation arrest of these follicles and premature luteinization leading to atresia. Under the effect of LH, theca cells proliferate and ultimately contribute to the stroma leading to stromal abundance. Theca cell population, thus, keeps on increasing every cycle, once PCOS starts manifesting itself. This manifestation is initiated with the metabolic derangement, especially involving insulin metabolism.

ANTRAL FOLLICLE COUNT IN POLYCYSTIC OVARY AND ITS HORMONAL IMPLICATIONS

Anti-Müllerian hormone (AMH) is a biomarker secreted from granulosa cells of small antral follicles and leads to follicular arrest in women with PCOS. AMH does not appear to be helpful for all subjects with PCOS but may be of some value in those who are anovulatory. However, FNPO was highly sensitive in all phenotypes, and was the single best criterion assessed for all subjects, suggesting the important role of ultrasound. AMH, obesity, insulin resistance (IR), and high androgen levels relate to large size of antral follicle pool and large ovarian volume (OV) in PCOS. Obesity and IR may enhance follicular excess by dysregulation of AMH through pathway of hyperandrogenemia.[16]

The mean FNPO of follicles 2–5 mm in size is significantly higher in polycystic ovaries than in controls, while it was similar within 6–9 mm range. Within 2–5 mm range, significant relationship was found between FNPO and androgens but FNPO in the range of 6–9 mm was significantly and negatively related to body mass index (BMI) and fasting serum insulin level.

ARRANGEMENT OF FOLLICLES

The antral and atretic follicles get arranged peripherally or are dispersed in the stroma, and thus may categorize polycystic ovary (PCO) as peripheral cystic pattern and general cystic pattern (GCP). In peripheral cystic pattern, there is typical garland-like arrangement of follicles and in GCP, the follicles can be seen throughout the ovary[17] **(Figs. 3A and B)**. Studies have documented that the ovary is multifollicular in adolescence. Because the androgen

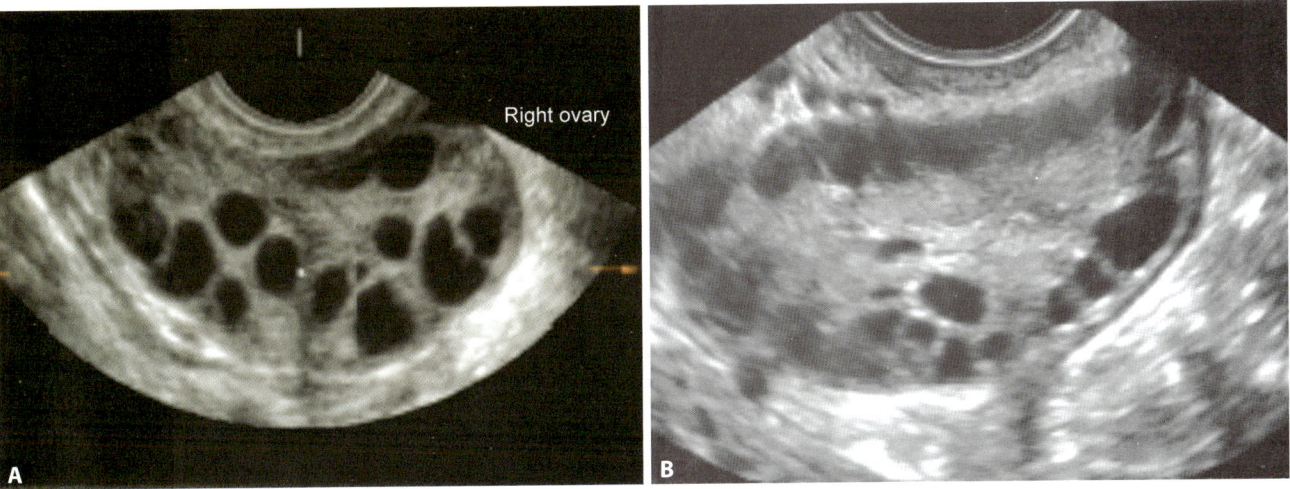

Figs. 3A and B: (A) Generalized polycystic pattern; (B) Peripheral polycystic pattern.

excess in the PCOS patients causes LH excess as a result of insulin derangement, this as a triggering factor leads to follicles exposure to LH, atresia, and theca cell proliferation, leading to stromal excess and generalized cystic polycystic ovary. If at this stage the metabolic derangement is not corrected, proliferation of theca cells and so stromal abundance keeps on increasing leading to either enlargement of the ovary first or pushing the follicles to the periphery to allow stromal expansion ultimately leading to peripheral cystic PCO.[18,19] So, multicystic ovary to generalized cystic PCO, to peripheral cystic PCO is a process of evolution of the disease. This indicates that the patients who have more severe form of disease or a long-standing disease have a peripheral cystic pattern and evidently will have worse hormonal milieu as compared to those who have generalized polycystic pattern.

STROMAL ABUNDANCE

Hyperdense stroma and stromal abundance have been described with polycystic ovaries since the first definition of the syndrome by Stein–Leventhal.

Stromal abundance can present as increased echogenicity because stroma is densely packed, and hence there is increased stromal area or increased stroma volume in large ovary. Patients having long-standing PCOS and long-standing anovulation have denser stroma. Most severe form of stromal abundance, hyperthecosis, presents large ovaries with almost absence of cystic lesions—solid-looking ovaries **(Fig. 4)**.

Polycystic ovaries show a hyperechoic stroma but assessment of this hyperechogenicity is subjective not only

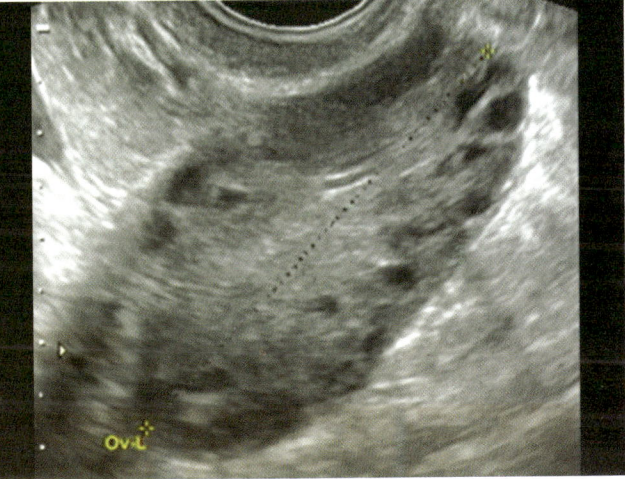

Fig. 4: Solid-looking polycystic ovary (PCO).

to the operator but also to equipment settings.[20,21] Though ovarian stroma can be stamped as hyperechoic when it is more echogenic than myometrium. This hyperechogenicity is especially useful for its differentiation from multicystic ovaries, which are normally seen in adolescence and have multiple follicles of variable sizes and nonhyperechogenic stroma. Increased stromal echogenicity for diagnosis of PCO has a sensitivity of 94% and specificity of 90%[22] **(Figs. 5A and B)**. Other studies have documented that stromal index (stromal echogenicity/total ovarian echogenicity) was significantly higher in PCOS than controls.[23]

Stromal abundance can be measured on ultrasound as stromal area in the most longitudinal section of ovary on 2D US. Stromal area of 4.6 cm^2 has 91% sensitivity and

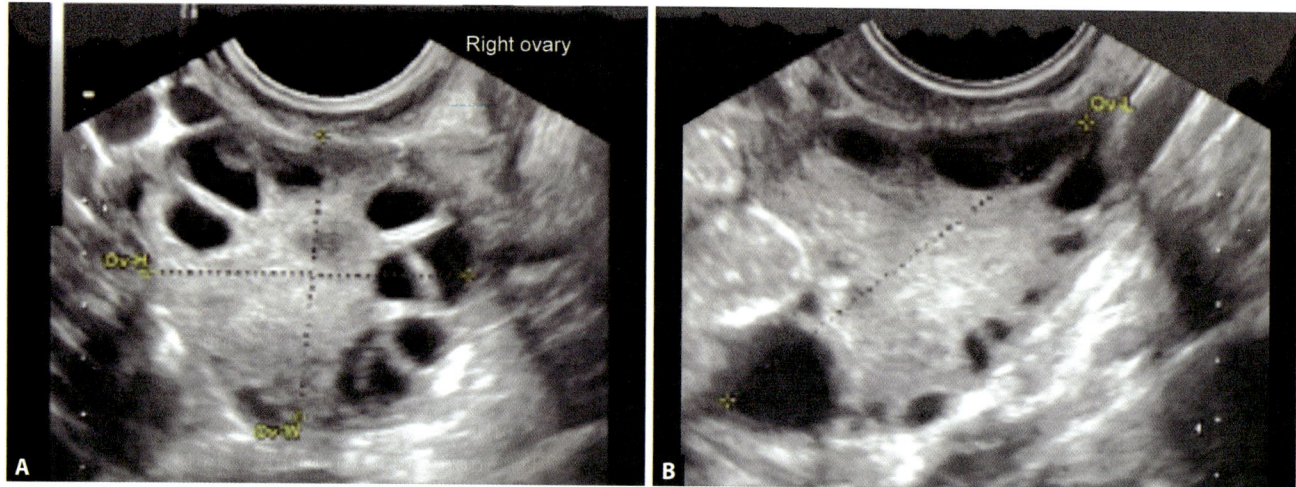

Figs. 5A and B: Dense hyperechoic stroma of polycystic ovary (PCO).

86% specificity for diagnosis of PCOS. The ovarian area can also be measured in this same section. Ovarian area of 5.3 cm^2 has 93% sensitivity and 91% specificity for diagnosis of PCOS.[7]

But the ratio of stromal area to ovarian area has been found to be more reliable. S/A (Stromal area/Ovarian area ratio) ratio also has a strong correlation with serum androgens (S androgens), especially testosterone and androstenedione, and insulin.[24] S/A ratio of 0.34 is diagnostic of PCOS and can be correlated with S. androstenedione.

Sensitivity for diagnosis of PCOS:
- Ovarian volume (13.21 cm^3) = 21%
- Ovarian area (7 cm^2) = 4%
- Stromal area (1.95 cm^2) = 62%
- Stromal/total area (0.34) = 100%

Mean stromal area/mean ovarian area ratio of 0.34 (**Fig. 6**) and above also has a specificity of 100% in the same study.[25]

STROMAL ABUNDANCE IN POLYCYSTIC OVARY AND ITS HORMONAL IMPLICATIONS

Hyperandrogenic subjects showed higher values of stromal area and S/A ratio, with no difference in OV and ovarian area.[4] S/A has also been found to be the best significant predictor of elevated androgen and testosterone levels. This parameter may be used in routine clinical practice for improving US diagnosis of PCOS.[25] Stromal abundance may be better assessed by stromal volume than with stromal area. Stromal volume can be assessed by using threshold volume on VOCAL calculated OV.

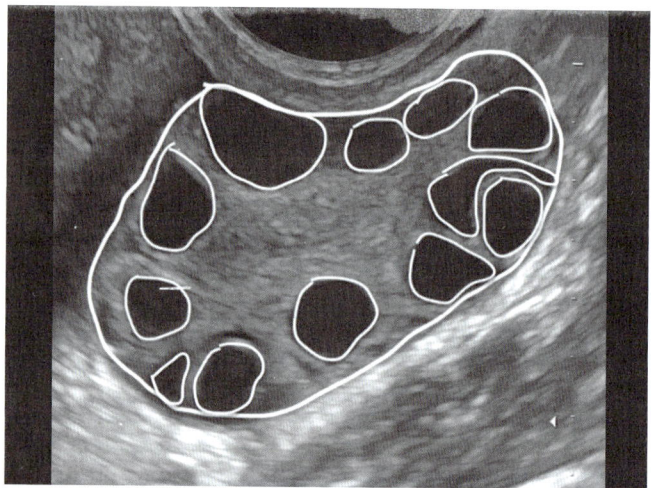

Fig. 6: B-mode ultrasound image of the ovary showing measurement of the ovarian area and follicular area to calculate stromal area.

The 3D US provides a new method for objective quantitative assessment of follicle count, OV, stromal volume, and blood flow in the ovary.[18] OV calculation by 3D US has been found to be useful over 2D evaluation of ovarian long diameter or volume by 2D US (**Fig. 7 and Table 1**).

Theca cells of PCOS women hyper-respond to gonadotropins (LH) and produce excess androgens. This is due to an escape of their normal downregulation to gonadotropins. This dysregulation is linked to excess of insulin and insulin-like growth factor-1 (IGF-1). Hyperinsulinemia is a key factor to the pathogenesis of PCOS. Insulin augments LH-stimulated androgen production by stromal cells. Androgen in turn causes proliferation of stromal and theca cells. This leads to

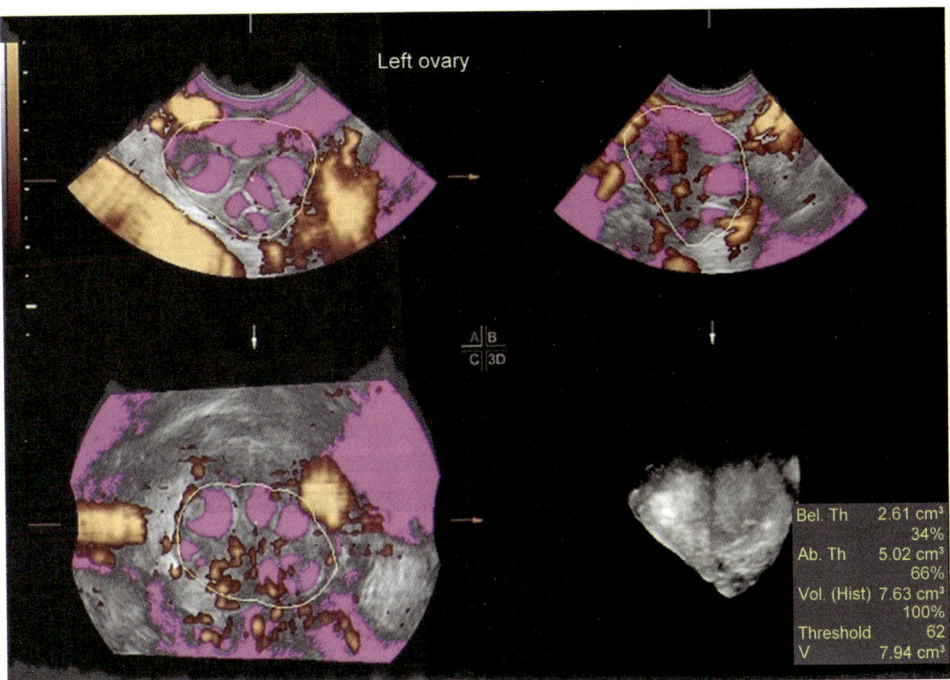

Fig. 7: 3D ultrasound with virtual organ computer-aided analysis (VOCAL) calculated volume of the ovary with threshold volume to calculate stromal volume.

TABLE 1: Left and right ovarian volume of normal versus polycystic ovaries.

Ovarian volume	Right	Left
Normal	5.3 ± 2.0 cc	5.7 ± 1.6 cm³
Polycystic ovarian disease (PCOD)	12.2 ± 4.7 cm³	10.5 ± 3.6 cm³ [23]

increased stroma in the PCO. Stromal volume was positively correlated with serum androstenedione concentrations in patients with PCOS.[26] Increased androstenedione secretion as shown earlier is due to hyperinsulinemia.[27]

When OVs and stromal volumes were compared and correlated with both fasting and postprandial (PP) insulin levels, a positive correlation was seen between OVs and stromal volumes and fasting and PP insulin levels.

With Pearson correlation significance level of 0.01 (2-tailed) the correlation for:
- OV to fasting insulin was 0.651
- OV to PP insulin was 0.409
- Stromal volume to fasting insulin was 0.736
- Stromal volume to PP insulin was 0.428

Stromal volumes and OVs and AFC correlated significantly well with the fasting insulin levels, more than with PP insulin levels in obese PCOS patients. It is the stromal volume that can be best correlated with fasting insulin levels followed by OVs and AFC.[28]

Pache et al. have shown that the degree of IR can be correlated with OV and stromal echogenicity.[27]

STROMAL VASCULARITY

Women with PCOS have increased stromal volume and vascularity. Even with same echogenicity, PCOS has more stromal flow. In PCOs, intraovarian stromal flow has moderate-to-low resistance with RI of 0.50–0.58.[29]

Elevated LH levels may be responsible for increased stromal vascularization due to neoangiogenesis, catecholaminergic stimulation, and leukocyte and cytokine activation. This vascularity is inversely related to LH/FSH ratio. Tonic secretion of LH in early follicular phase in PCOS is also associated with theca and stromal cell hyperplasia and consequent androgen production leading to vasoconstrictive effect on the uterine arteries. Uterine artery pulsatility index (PI) is more than three and sometimes the diastolic flow is absolutely absent. Even in later phases of the cycle this effect continues. This leads to inadequate perfusion of the endometrium and is thought to be responsible for blastocyst implantation failure and high abortion rate in PCOS.

Looking at the hormonal correlation with the Doppler findings, it is evident that in patients in whom the hormonal milieu is worse, the Doppler findings are more

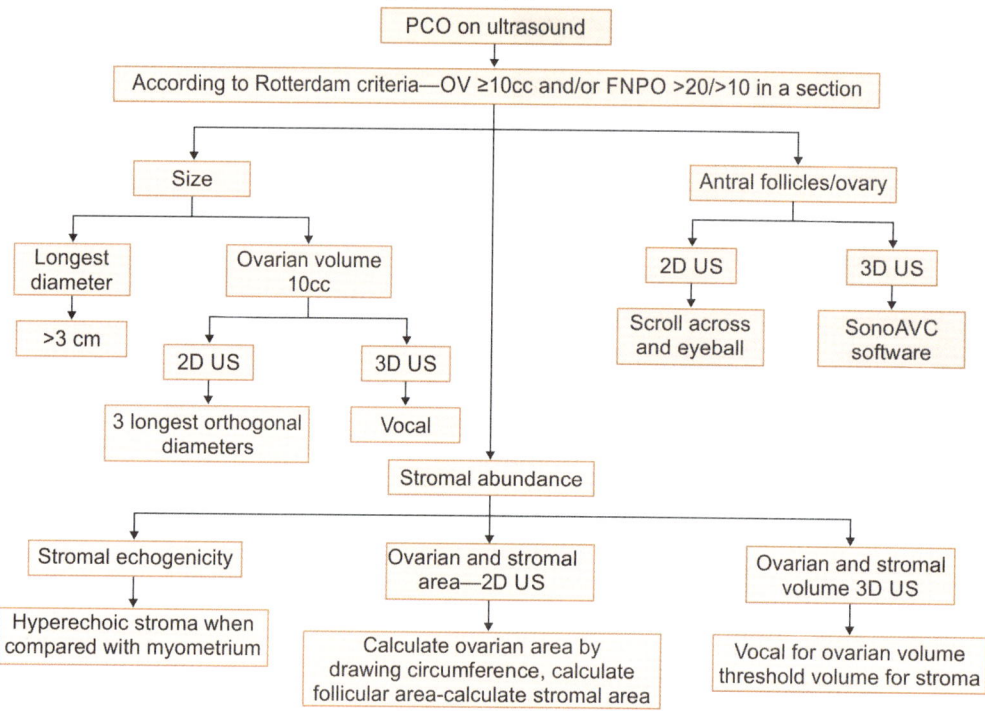

Flowchart 1: Polycystic ovary syndrome on ultrasound.

(2D US: two-dimensional ultrasound; 3D US: three-dimensional ultrasound; FNPO: follicle number per ovary; OV: ovarian volume; PCOS: polycystic ovarian syndrome; SonoAVC: sonography-based automated volume count; VOCAL: virtual organ computer-aided analysis)

prominent. As discussed earlier, the peripheral cystic pattern of PCO is an advanced stage then GCP, and so the intraovarian vascularity and uterine artery resistance are more in peripheral PCOs than in generalized PCOs.[30] Stromal vascularity is significantly higher in women with PCOS who are hyperandrogenic and lean rather than normoandrogenic and obese.[31] Fertile controls and PCOS women had similar total ovarian 3D power Doppler flow indices. Normal weight PCOS women had significantly higher total ovarian 3D power Doppler flow indices than their overweight counterparts.[32] Higher age, obesity, and amenorrhea as compared to young age, normal weight, and oligomenorrhea show higher uterine artery resistance and increased ovarian stromal flow. These are the patients who also have higher LH, higher androstenedione levels, and higher OVs.

Women with PCOS have higher stromal vascularization [vascularization index (VI) 3.85% vs. 2.79% and vascularization flow index (VFI) 1.27 vs. 0.85]. Though 2D power Doppler indices were not higher in PCOS than in controls.[33]

CONCLUSION

Ultrasound plays a major role **(Flowchart 1)** in not only diagnosis of PCOs, but also helps to understand the pathophysiology, variable presentation of the syndrome, and variable response of the patients to ovulation induction.

REFERENCES

1. Thatcher. Defining PCOS—a perspective: The American Infertility Association Newsletter; 2001.
2. Rotterdam ESHRE/ASRM-sponsored PCOS consensus workshop group. Revised 2003 consensus on diagnostic criteria and long-term health risks related to polycystic ovary syndrome (PCOS). Hum Reprod. 2004;19(1):41-7.
3. Takahashi K, Eda Y, Abu Musa A, Okada S, Yoshino K, Kitao M. Transvaginal ultrasound imaging, histopathology and endocrinopathy in patients with polycystic ovarian syndrome. Hum Reprod. 1994;9(7):1231-6.
4. Jonard S, Robert Y, Dewailly D. Revisiting the ovarian volume as a diagnostic criterion for polycystic ovaries. Hum Reprod. 2005;20(10):2893-8.
5. Allemand MC, Tummon IS, Phy JL, Foong SC, Dumesic DA, Session DR. Diagnosis of polycystic ovaries by three-dimensional transvaginal ultrasound. Fertil Steril. 2006;85(1):214-9.
6. Kyei-Mensah AA, Lin Tan S, Zaidi J, Jacobs HS. Relationship of ovarian stromal volume to serum androgen concentrations in patients with polycystic ovary syndrome. Hum Reprod. 1998;13(6):1437-41.

7. Wu MH, Tang HH, Hsu CC, Wang ST, Huang KE. The role of three-dimensional ultrasonographic images in ovarian measurement. Fertil Steril. 1998;69(6):1152-5.
8. Legro RS, Gnatuk CL, Kunselman AR, Dunaif A. Changes in glucose tolerance over time in women with polycystic ovary syndrome: A controlled study. J Clin Endocrinol Metab. 2005;90(6):3236-42.
9. Jonard S, Robert Y, Cortet-Rudelli C, Decanter C, Dewailly D, Pigny P. Ultrasound examination of polycystic ovaries: Is it worth counting the follicles? Hum Reprod. 2003;18(3):598-603.
10. Kim HJ, Adams JM, Gudmundson JA, Arason G, Pau CT, Welt CK. Polycystic ovary morphology: Age-based ultrasound criteria. Fertil Steril. 2017;108(3):548-53.
11. Dewailly D, Gronier H, Poncelet E, Robin G, Leroy M, Pigny P, et al. Diagnosis of polycystic ovarian syndrome (PCOS): Revisiting the threshold values of follicle count on ultrasound and of the serum AMH level for the definition of polycystic ovaries. Hum Reprod. 2011;26(11):3123-9.
12. Lujan ME, Jarrett BY, Brooks ED, Reines JK, Peppin AK, Muhn N, et al. Updated ultrasound criteria for polycystic ovary syndrome: Reliable thresholds for elevated follicle population and ovarian volume. Hum Reprod. 2013;28(5):1361-8.
13. Balen AH, Laven JS, Tan SL, Dewailly D. Ultrasound assessment of the polycystic ovary: International consensus definitions. Hum Reprod Update. 2003;9(6):505-14.
14. Chen Y, Li L, Chen X, Zhang Q, Wang W, Li Y, et al. Ovarian volume and follicle number in the diagnosis of polycystic ovary syndrome in Chinese women. Ultrasound Obstet Gynecol. 2008;32:700-3.
15. Köşüş N, Köşüş A, Turhan NÖ, Kamalak Z. Do threshold values of ovarian volume and follicle number for diagnosing polycystic ovarian syndrome in Turkish women differ from western countries? Eur J Obstet Gynecol Reprod Biol. 2011;154(2):177-81.
16. Chen MJ, Yang WS, Chen CL, Wu MY, Yang YS, Ho HN. The relationship between anti-Müllerian hormone, androgen and insulin resistance on the number of antral follicles in women with polycystic ovary syndrome. Hum Reprod. 2008;23(4):952-7.
17. Matsunaga I, Hata T, Kitao M. Ultrasonographic identification of polycystic ovary. Asia Oceania J Obstet Gynecol. 1985;11(2):227-32.
18. Ardaens Y, Robert Y, Lemaitre L, Fossati P, Dewailly D. Polycystic ovarian disease: Contribution of transvaginal endosonography and reassessment of ultrasonographic diagnosis. Fertil Steril. 1991;55(6):1062-8.
19. Robert Y, Dubrulle F, Gaillandre L, Ardaens Y, Thomas-Desrousseaux P, Lemaitre L, et al. Ultrasound assessment of ovarian stroma hypertrophy in hyperandrogenism and ovulation disorders: Visual analysis versus computerized quantification. Fertil Steril. 1995;64(2):307-12.
20. Pache TD, Wladimiroff JW, Hop WC, Fauser BC. How to discriminate between normal and polycystic ovaries: Transvaginal US study. Radiology. 1992;183(2):421-3.
21. Buckett WM, Bouzayen R, Watkin KL, Tulandi T, Tan SL. Ovarian stromal echogenicity in women with normal and polycystic ovaries. Hum Reprod. 1999;14(3):618-21.
22. Dewailly D, Robert Y, Helin I, Ardaens Y, Thomas-Desrousseaux P, Lemaitre L, et al. Ovarian stromal hypertrophy in hyperandrogenic women. Clin Endocrinol (Oxf). 1994;41(5):557-62.
23. Belosi C, Selvaggi L, Apa R, Guido M, Romualdi D, Fulghesu AM, et al. Is the PCOS diagnosis solved by ESHRE/ASRM 2003 consensus or could it include ultrasound examination of the ovarian stroma? Hum Reprod. 2006;21(12):3108-15.
24. Fulghesu AM, Ciampelli M, Belosi C, Apa R, Pavone V, Lanzone A. A new ultrasound criterion for the diagnosis of polycystic ovary syndrome: The ovarian stroma/total area ratio. Fertil Steril. 2001;76(2):326-31.
25. Fulghesu AM, Angioni S, Frau E, Belosi C, Apa R, Mioni R, et al. Ultrasound in polycystic ovary syndrome-the measuring of ovarian stroma and relationship with circulating androgens: Results of multicentric study. Hum Reprod. 2007;22(9):2501-8.
26. Balen A, Conway G, Homburg R, Legro R. Polycystic ovary syndrome: A guide to clinical management, first edition. London: Taylor & Francis Group; 2013
27. Pache TD, de Jong FH, Hop WC, Fauser BC. Association between ovarian changes assessed by transvaginal sonography and clinical and endocrine signs of polycystic ovary syndrome. Feril Steril. 1993;59:544-9.
28. Nagori CB, Panchal SY. Assessing correlation between ovarian and stromal volumes and fasting and postprandial insulin levels in PCOS patients. Presented at ISUOG, Chicago; 2008.
29. Battalgia C, Artini PG, D'Ambrogio G, Genazzani A, D Genazzani AR. The role of color Doppler imaging in the diagnosis of polycystic ovarian syndrome. Am J Obstet Gynecol. 1995;172:108-13.
30. Battalgia C, Artini PG, Salvatori M, Giulini S, Petraglia F, Maxia N. Ultrasonographic patterns of polycystic ovaries: Color Doppler and hormonal correlations. Ultrasound Obstet Gynecol. 1998;11(5):332-6.
31. Ozkan S, Vural B, Caliskan E, Bodur H, Turkoz E, Vural F. Color Doppler sonographic analysis of uterine and ovarian artery blood flow in women with polycystic ovary syndrome. J Clin Ultrasound. 2007;35(6):305-13.
32. Ng EH, Chan CC, Yeung WS, Ho PC. Comparison of ovarian stromal blood flow between fertile women with normal ovaries and infertile women with polycystic ovary syndrome. Hum Reprod. 2005;20(7):1881-6.
33. Lam PM, Jhonson IR, Rainne-Fenning NJ. Three-dimensional ultrasound features of the polycystic ovary and the effect of different phenotypic expressions on these parameters. Hum Reprod. 2007;22(12):3116-23.

Oocyte Retrieval

Chapter 24

INTRODUCTION

Oocyte retrieval is aspiration of mature follicles to retrieve oocytes and is the primary requirement for the in vitro fertilization (IVF) procedures.

Lenz et al. first described percutaneous transabdominal (TA)/transvesical aspiration of follicles under ultrasound (US) guidance in 1981.[1] In 1982, transvaginal (TV) oocyte retrieval with TA US guidance was described.[2] TV ovum retrieval with TV US guidance with mechanical TV sector scanner was first described by Kemeter and Feichtinger in the late 1980s[3] **(Fig. 1)**. This was a major breakthrough in IVF treatment and was soon universally accepted. TV oocyte retrieval is a very simple and well-accepted method with very low complication rate.

CURRENT METHOD

The method used currently is TV US-guided TV oocyte retrieval.

Preprocedure **(Flowchart 1)**: Administration of an intravenous bolus of antibiotics for women with history of severe pelvic inflammatory disease or if an endometrioma is punctured. In the Indian subcontinent, antibiotics are routinely administered.

Premedication and anesthesia **(Flowchart 1)**: Provide effective anesthesia and analgesia for TV oocyte retrieval as it is painful. But also remember, no technique of anesthesia, analgesia, or sedation is free from side effects. So, adhere to recognized standards of practice. Therefore, as little as possible should be the rule. Conscious sedation is a safe and acceptable method of providing analgesia. In most centers, short general anesthesia is preferred. Intravenous fentanyl, propofol, and midazolam are the commonly used medications and do not affect the outcome of IVF. Paracervical or preovarian blocks may be used. For paracervical blocks, a local anesthetic is injected into 2–6 sites at a depth of 3–7 mm alongside the vaginal portion of the cervix in the vaginal fornices. Some centers also use hypnotism for analgesia.

Technique

All sterile precautions are taken; from washing hands to wearing a sterile gown. Only powder-free sterile gloves are used. The trolley for the procedure should contain the painting and draping requirements, a Sims speculum, an anterior retractor, and an Allis forceps, in cases of unexpected bleeding or minor complications.

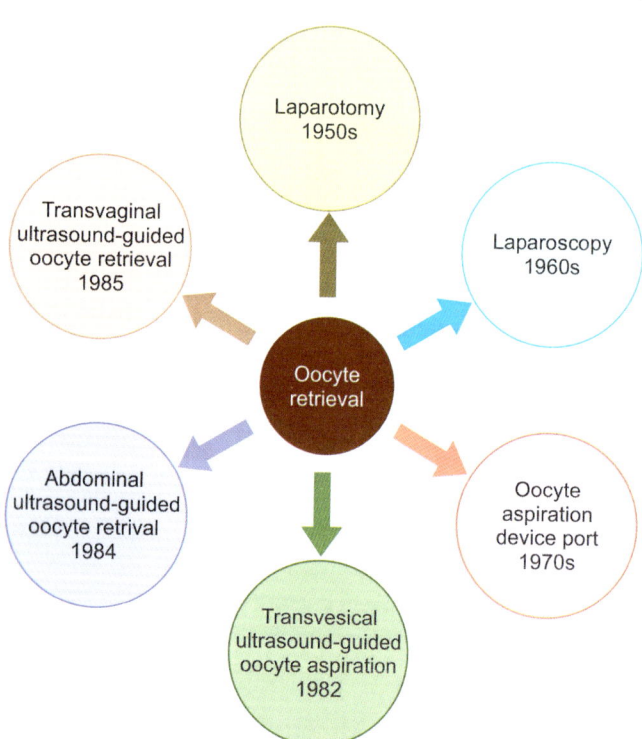

Fig. 1: History of evolvement of the current ovum retrieval technique.

Flowchart 1: Preprocedure preparation for oocyte retrieval.

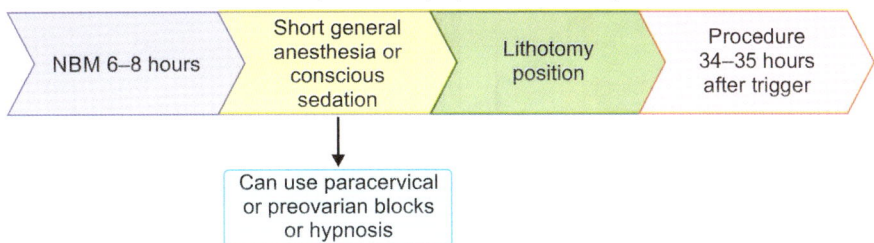

NBM: nothing by mouth

The disposables include a sterilized probe cover and a sterilized condom without spermicidal gel. A biopsy guide is absolutely essential.

Vagina is cleaned thoroughly with normal saline and not antiseptics.

One may use culture medium to cleanse the vagina. It is essential to clean the probe with the special probe cleansing solutions provided by the manufacturers before the procedure. The US transducer is enclosed in sterile condom or a plastic sleeve with US gel or saline inside **(Fig. 2)**, prior to insertion into the vagina. Probe should be thoroughly cleaned with a damp cloth after each procedure. The biopsy guide is fixed on the probe. Place the probe in the vagina to assess the endometrial thickness, position and accessibility of the ovaries, and the number of follicles to be aspirated. Switch on the biopsy guide on the screen. The guide helps to identify the position of the needle and the path it will take when the needle is advanced through the vaginal fornix into the ovary.

The transducer should be so positioned that the ovary is placed closest possible to the needle tip. Transducer is then manipulated to bring the follicles one after the other on the biopsy guide with minimum possible probe movement as these are punctured serially. This is to minimize the damage to the ovarian stroma.

Needles (Flowchart 2, Figs. 3 and 4)

The needle is connected to a test tube, prewarmed at 37°C in hot blocks by tubing and suction is applied either from a foot-operated pump **(Figs. 3A and B)** or manually. Before aspiration, the needle and the tubing are flushed with flushing medium.

Medium with heparin is used for this purpose. This prevents clotting of blood in the tubing that may be aspirated along with the follicular fluid. Needle is advanced from the vagina into the ovary under ultrasound guidance.

A follicle aspiration equipment is shown in **Figure 5**.

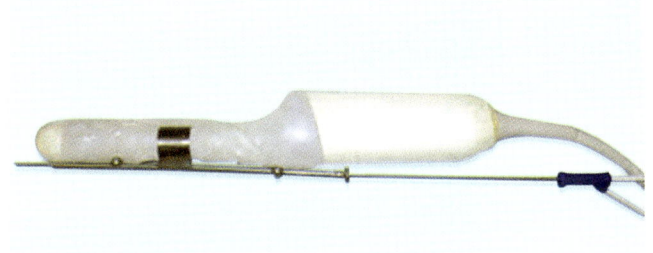

Fig. 2: Vaginal ultrasound transducer covered with sterile condom with needle guide attached. The needle tip is protruding from the proximal end of the probe.

Flowchart 2: Oocyte retrieval needle requirements.

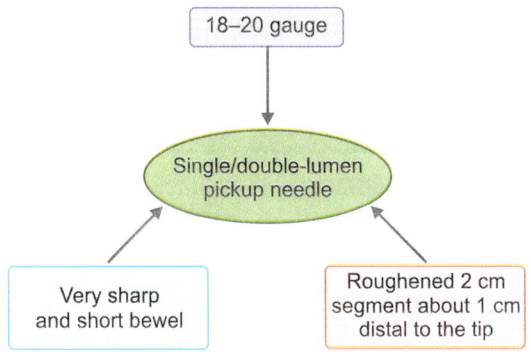

Needle path is usually at 2 o'clock position for puncturing the left ovary and 10 o'clock position for left ovary in the vagina, lateral to the cervix **(Fig. 6)**. But when ovaries are fixed or positioned high up in the pelvis, the path may have to be changed. If possible, the follicle should be punctured from the side of the ovary, with an aim to induce minimal damage to the ovary. As far as possible, only single vaginal puncture with one or two ovarian punctures maximum should be done on each side. This approach reduces the risk of bleeding.

Entering the ovary may be difficult in mobile ovary and then pressure on the abdomen may be required to fix the ovaries. Find the nearest leading follicle and then

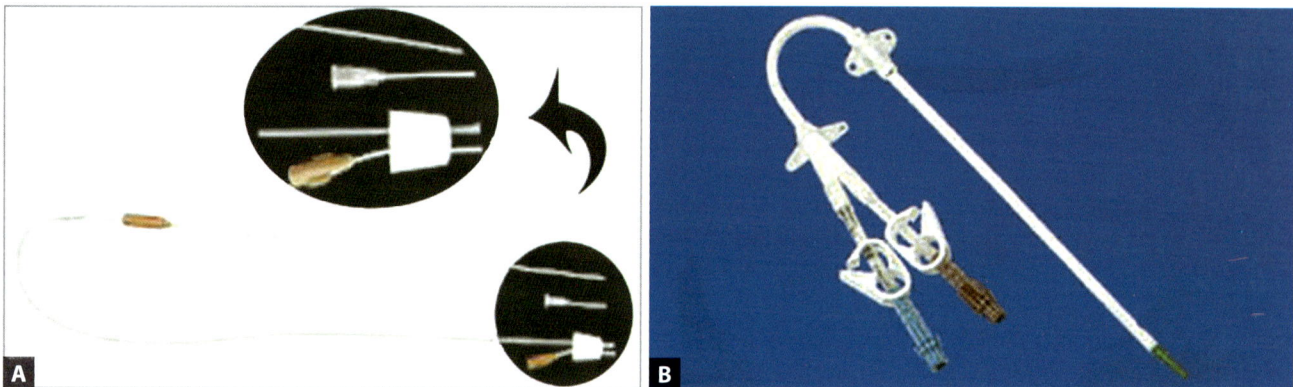

Figs. 3A and B: (A) Single-lumen ovum pickup needle with the connections in the cock to fit into the test tube and to be attached to the suction machine; (B) Double-lumen suction catheter for ovum pickup.

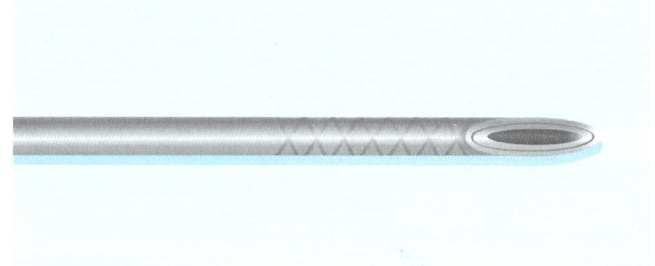

Fig. 4: Needle tip of the ovum pickup needle. The markings close to the tip make the surface rough and therefore make the needle easily visible on ultrasound.

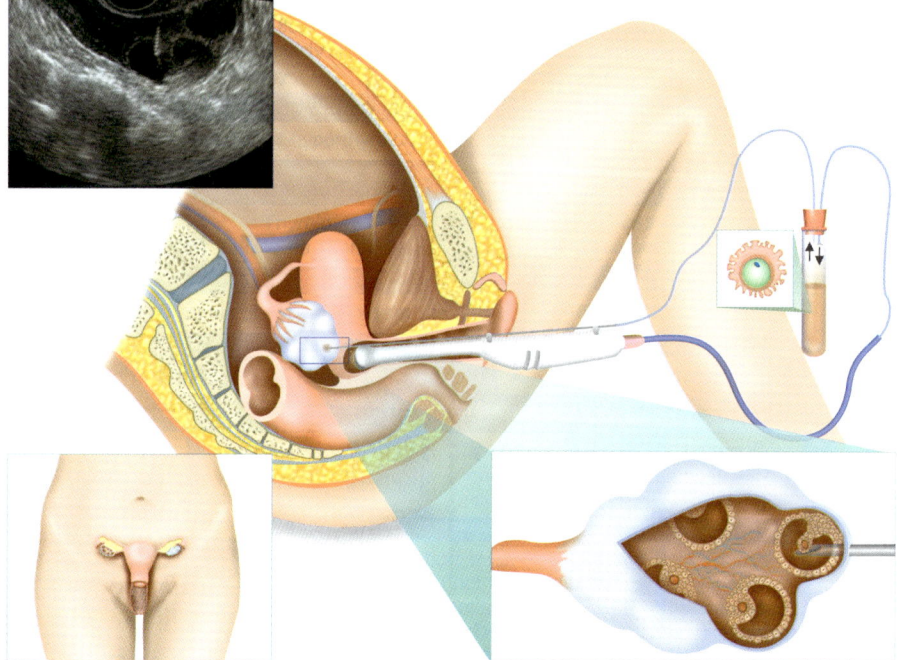

Fig. 5: Follicle aspiration equipment. An assembled follicle aspiration single-lumen needle connected to a test tube. The test tube is in turn connected to a suction pump. The needle is attached to the transvaginal ultrasound transducer through needle guide and bracket.

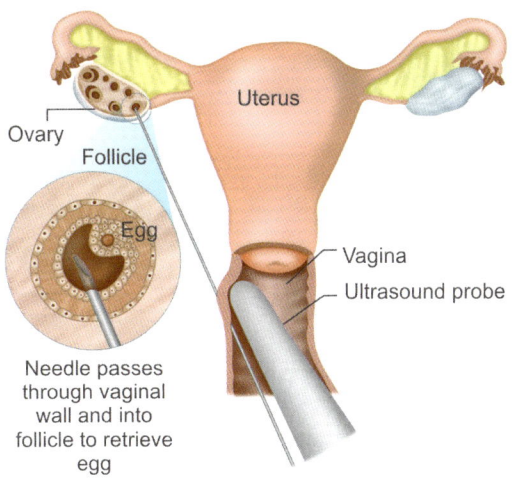

Fig. 6: Needle path during ovum pickup from its site of entry from the vaginal walls to its entry into the ovary.

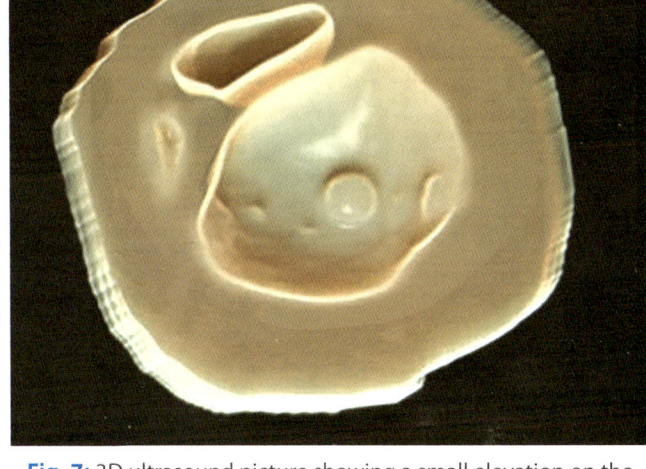

Fig. 7: 3D ultrasound picture showing a small elevation on the follicle wall, this is cumulus.

needle must be advanced firmly and quickly into the follicle. Ensure that the needle tip is correctly positioned at the center of the follicle and then the negative pressure is applied. Negative pressure of 110–120 mm Hg is required.

Always confirm that you are puncturing the follicle and not the vessel by manipulating the probe to view the follicle in sagittal and transverse plane and if in doubt, use Doppler.

Gentle rotation of the needle helps to suck the ovum, if stuck, from all the walls of the follicle. Contents are aspirated till the follicle is empty. The next follicle is entered without withdrawing the needle out of the ovary, if in the same path. Keep needle in the ovary and aspirate several follicles one after another with careful gentle manipulation. The order of aspiration of different follicles should be such that the needle manipulation is the least.

Flushing is recommended only if there are very few follicles and especially when the cumulus (**Fig. 7**) has been demonstrated in the follicle on pretrigger scan and oocyte is not retrieved from that follicle (**Fig. 5**). All follicles till 10–12 mm size are aspirated as at times even a 10-mm sized follicle may reveal a fertilizable follicle in aspirate.

Bowels in the path of the needle can be removed by rotating and pushing movements of the probe. At times, one may have to pass the needle through the uterus to access the ovary, but in such cases, one needs to ensure that vessels are avoided. After completing aspiration of all the follicles, repeat the entire procedure for the opposite ovary and then remove the probe. Put the speculum and check for the bleeding from the puncture site. If required, apply pressure with a sterilized gauze for a few minutes to stop bleeding. Rarely, a vaginal pack may be required for a few minutes to control bleeding.

It is best not to puncture hydrosalpinx (**Fig. 8A**) or endometriomas (**Fig. 8B**), while doing oocyte retrieval. However, if a hydrosalpinx or an endometrioma is punctured inadvertently, prophylactic antibiotic, preferably intravenous, must be administered.

The TA route of ultrasound guidance and puncture may be needed rarely for oocyte retrieval when ovary is not approachable from vaginal route; if it is placed high up in the pelvis, as in patients with absent uterus; or if the patient has had vaginoplasty. Though none of these are absolute indications for TA oocyte retrieval as it depends on the operators' convenience and expertise for TV approach.

Complications

Generally, very few technical difficulties are encountered during vaginal egg collections. The main risks of TV oocyte recovery are pelvic infection (0.6%) and bleeding (>100 mL in 0.8% cases), which may be serious, sometimes even fatal. Appropriate preoperative vaginal preparation and minimizing the number of repeated vaginal penetrations may serve to lower the risk of infection (**Flowchart 3**).

Intestinal, vascular, uterine, and tubal injuries with the aspiration needle have also been reported. Bleeding and infections may be serious and sometimes, even have fatal complications.

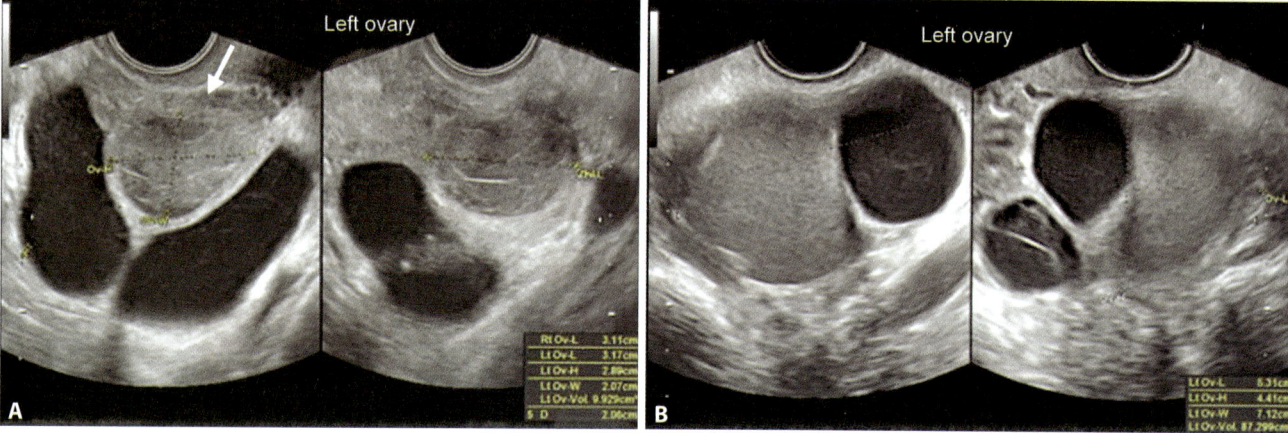

Figs. 8A and B: (A) B-mode ultrasound image of an ovary containing corpus luteum (arrow) and an anechoic sausage-shaped lesion surrounding it from below, which is a hydrosalpinx; (B) B-mode ultrasound image of ovary showing two cystic structures—one that is anechoic appears to be a follicle and the other with low-level echogenicity is most likely an endometrioma.

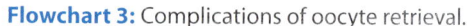

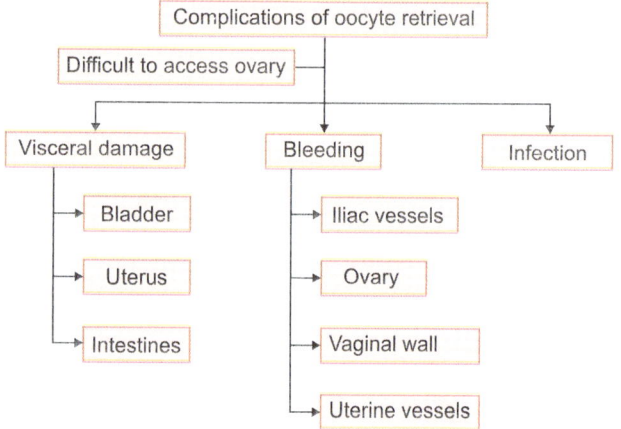

Flowchart 3: Complications of oocyte retrieval.

Ovaries are located close to the iliac vessels, and therefore iliac vessels are vulnerable to injury during ovum pickup by inexperienced hands. Care must always be taken when aspirating the follicles that are close to major vessels (internal iliac vessels). Another possible site of bleeding is from the vaginal wall. This is especially common when there is congestion of the vaginal wall. This bleeding is never severe, though may be frightening for the patient. It stops by manual pressure on the bleeding site for a few minutes or by tamponing. The third possible site from where the bleeding would occur is uterine vessels. This happens when the ovary is adherent to the uterus and placed high up in the pelvis. This can be prevented by carefully managing the needle path.

Ovum Pickup

The process of oocyte retrieval can be summarized in the following steps:
- Administer IV general anesthesia or local anesthesia and sedation
- Consider antibiotic cover
- Aseptic technique is a must
- Lithotomy position of the patient, clean and drape
- Cleanse TV probe and cover it with sterile cover and condom with or without gel
- Set biopsy guide on scanner and fix the biopsy guide on the probe
- Introduce the probe to image the ovary in alignment with the biopsy line
- Introduce the pickup needle through fornix
- Apply suction as the follicle is punctured
- Aspirate all follicles one after the other and repeat for the other ovary
- Remove probe and check for bleeding

REFERENCES

1. Lenz S, Lauritsen JG, Kjellow M. Collection of human oocytes for in vitro fertilization by sonographically guided follicular puncture. Lancet. 1981;23:1163.
2. Lenz S, Lauristen JG. Ultrasonically guided percutaneous aspiration of human follicles under local anesthesia: a new method of collecting oocytes for in vitro fertilization. Fertil Steril. 1982;38:673-7.
3. Feichtinger W, Kemeter P. Transvaginal sector can sonography for needle guided transvaginal follicle aspiration and other applications in gynecologic routine and research. Fertil Steril. 1986;45:722-5.

Embryo Transfer

INTRODUCTION

Embryo transfer (ET) is a critical step in determining the final outcome of in vitro fertilization (IVF) treatment. Though evidently simple, this procedure demands a lot of perfection and precision. It is a true blend of science and art. Optimizing the technique of ET would provide the best chance of pregnancy **(Box 1)**.

TECHNIQUE

- Pretransfer ultrasound is done to check uterocervical curvature and uterocervical length. The length of the uterus is measured from the fundal end of the endometrium to external os **(Fig. 1)**.
- Asepsis is very essential. Patient lies in lithotomy position. Vagina is cleaned with warm normal saline. Gauze soaked in normal saline is used to wipe off all the vaginal secretions. Cusco's speculum is commonly used to visualize the cervix with minimal manipulation to cervix and uterus. Some units use Sim's speculum and Allis forceps or tenaculum to visualize the cervix and straighten the uterocervical canal to make the ET easier. Embryo-loaded catheter is brought to the transfer room only when everything is set. Keep the theater lights dimmed when ET catheter is brought to the operation theater. It is also essential to maintain the room temperature at 27–29°C. Introduce the transfer catheter into the cervix, under transabdominal ultrasound guidance. If uterocervical canal on pretransfer ultrasound is not straight, one may electively use a stiff outer sheath or a cervical cannula for introduction of the transfer catheter through it. In any case, the embryo is not retained in the catheter for more than 2 minutes. If it takes longer, the embryos are replaced back into the culture dish and reloaded later. Double-sheathed ET catheter is to be used in such cases. After introducing the outer sheath, which is firm in consistency, its position is confirmed beyond the internal os. The inner cannula is introduced through this sheath later on. Cannula tip is placed 1–1.5 cm caudal from the fundus of the uterus. Transfer is done in 15–25 µL of medium. Larger volume may lead to lower pregnancy rates, as this fluid may either flow out of the uterus or may fill up the tubes. Once the cannula is placed the desired level in the uterus, the piston of the syringe is pushed to inject fluid-containing embryos into the uterus. The ET cannula is seen as an echogenic line and can be traced from the internal os into the endometrial cavity and the tip is placed at least 1 cm proximal to the fundal end of

> **BOX 1:** Embryo transfer technique.
>
> *Embryo transfer can be optimized by:*
> - Pretransfer assessment of uterine cavity and cervical canal
> - Thorough and gentle removal of cervical mucus
> - *Avoid touching the uterine fundus to:*
>   – Avoid endometrial damage
>   – Avoid initiation of uterine contractions
> - *Confirm proper delivery of embryos inside the uterine cavity; this can be done by*:
>   – Confirming the location of catheter tip
>   – Visualize the easy passage of drop of media containing embryos followed by air bubble in the endometrial cavity

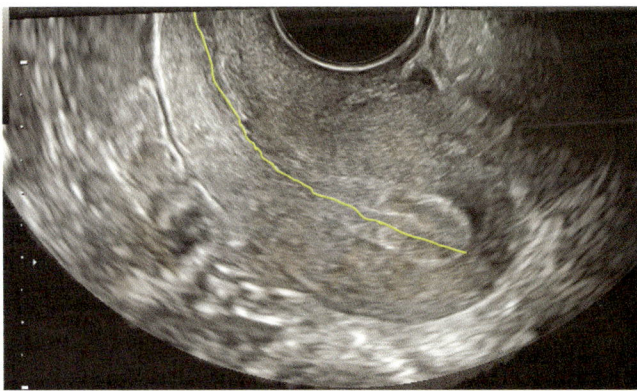

Fig. 1: Measuring the functional uterocervical length for embryo transfer.

the endometrium. The passage of embryos with the air bubble is seen as a release of echogenic spot into the endometrial cavity and is also known as "bullet sign" **(Figs. 2A to C)**. Then, the cannula is steadily held in position for a few seconds. After that, it is gently pulled out with the piston pressed not to cause a suction action. Fluid remaining in the cannula is checked under the microscope to confirm that embryos are not remaining in the cannula. Uterine contractions, expulsion of embryos, blood or mucus on the catheter tip, bacterial contamination of catheter, and retained embryos have all been associated with difficult ETs.

- Patients may be gently shifted into the bed and allowed to rest for 20–30 minutes. Success rates are similar regardless of the time for which the patient is kept motionless.
- Ease of ET and the time taken from taking out the embryo from the incubator to transferring it into the womb are the two most consistent factors that affect conception rates.

SUBOPTIMAL EMBRYO TRANSFERS

- When the cannula tip cannot be traced right till the midcavity and the embryos are released (Poor scanning skills or poor visibility due to patient's habitus, scars, excessive fat on abdomen, or uterine abnormalities)
- When after the release of the embryos, these are seen to float toward the midcavity from the release site; this may indicate more fluid in the cannula.
- Difficult to negotiate the cannula beyond internal os, which may be due to scar, abnormal curvature of endometrial cavity, or false passage.

In these cases, ultrasound guidance is useful to guide the catheter tip or the outer cannula in correct direction and help transferring the embryos to the correct site. This can be done by correcting the uterocervical angulation by manipulating and pulling the cervix with Allis forceps under ultrasound guidance or by using firm outer cannula to negotiate the difficult curvature.

Ultrasound guidance in this procedure has shown advantage over clinical touch or blind ET by significantly

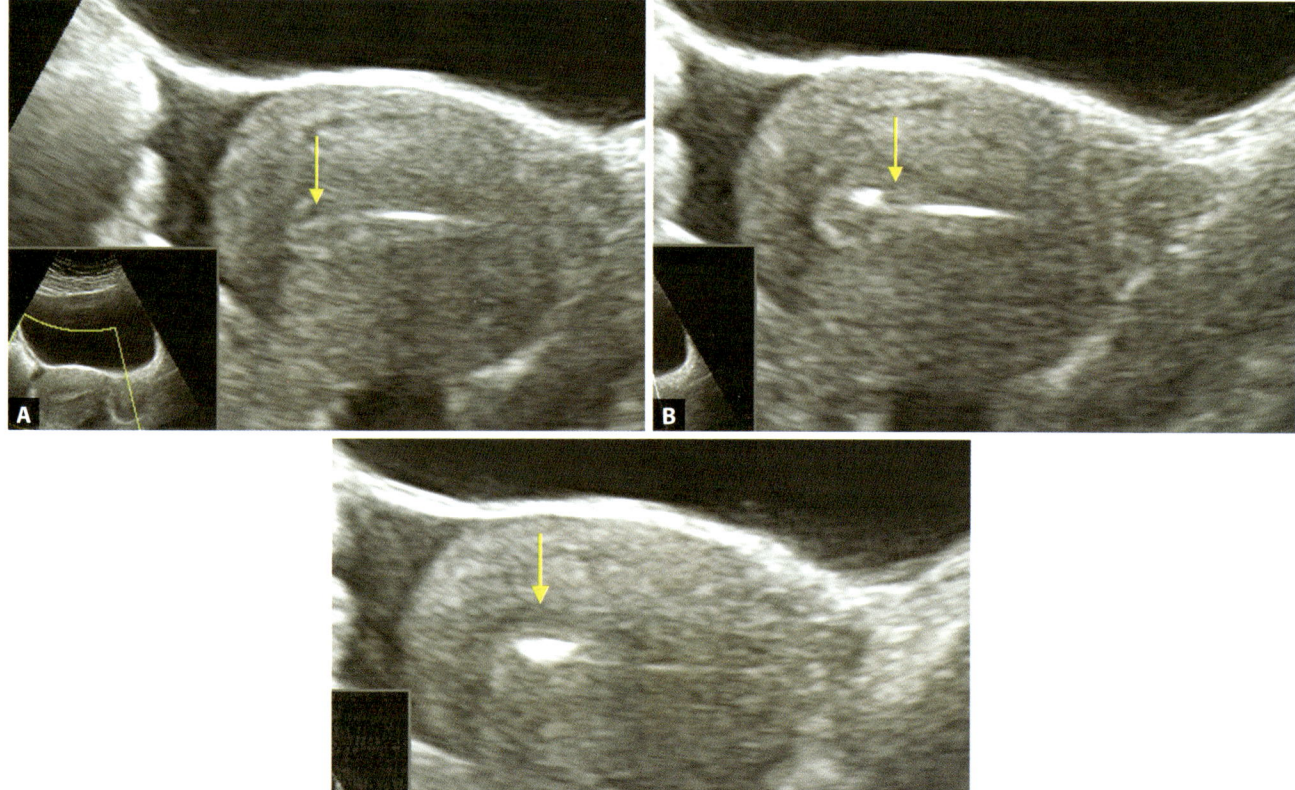

Figs. 2A to C: Embryo transfer. (A) Advancing the cannula in the uterus (arrows); (B) Releasing the embryo bubble in the uterus (arrows); (C) Retained embryo bubble in uterine cavity after removal of cannula (arrow).

increasing the chance of embryo implantation, ongoing pregnancy, and live birth due to the ease of transfer.[1,2]

In an exhaustive Cochrane database systematic review that included 13/15 randomized controlled trials, Brown et al.[1] reported significantly higher live birth/ongoing pregnancies per woman associated with ultrasound-guided ET (452/1376 compared with 353/1338) for clinical touch, or 1.40, 95% confidence interval (CI) 1.18–1.66 ($P <0.001$) in 6 studies.

Studies have shown that no significant changes in results have been observed whether transabdominal or transvaginal ultrasound is used for guidance.[3] However, transabdominal ultrasound is preferred as it does not interfere with the transvaginal or transcervical procedure of ET.

Ultrasound-guided ET enables the visualization of:[4]
- Guiding cannula and transfer catheter placement in relation to the endometrial surface and uterine fundus during ET
- The position and movement of a transfer-associated air bubble
- The impact of subendometrial–myometrial contractions leading to endometrial movement

ADVANTAGES OF ULTRASOUND-GUIDED EMBRYO TRANSFER

- Helps optimal placement of soft catheters
- Confirms that the catheter is beyond the internal os in cases of elongated cervical canal.
- Allows to guide the direction of the catheter along the contour of the endometrial cavity, especially in uteri with acute curves.
- Prevents damage to endometrium and plugging of catheter.
- Full bladder that is required for transabdominal ultrasound and that straightens the uterocervical angle and helps catheter passage.
- Helps to negotiate the catheter through difficult cervical canal.
- Helps to correct position of catheter tip for embryo deposition [point of maximum implantation potential (MIP)].

Ultrasound also has a role to ascertain the transfer at the point of MIP.

A large observational retrospective study by Gergely et al. has shown that if point of MIP is individually found in each patient with the help of three-dimensional (3D) ultrasound and embryos are deposited at this point, it can improve the implantation rates.[5] Point of MIP can be calculated by 3D ultrasound. On coronal section of the uterus, two lines are drawn, one on each side parallel to the cornu. The point at which these lines intersect is the point of MIP **(Fig. 3)**.

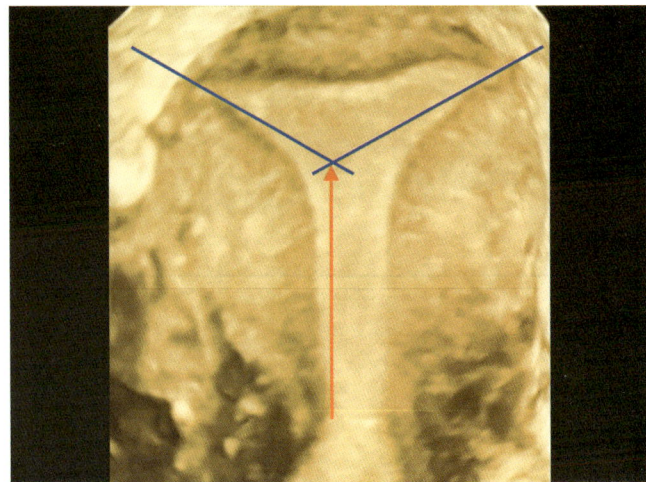

Fig. 3: Intersection of the lines drawn through the uterine cornu indicates the point of maximum implantation.

The use of ultrasound-guided transfer avoided tubal transfer in 7.4% of transfers. In a randomized trial, the use of transabdominal ultrasound guidance during ET improved the pregnancy rate from 33.7% to 50%.[6] In another retrospective study,[7] the pregnancy rate improved from 25% to 38% by using ultrasound during ET.

REFERENCES

1. Brown J, Buckingham K, Buckett W, Abou-Setta AM. Ultrasound versus "clinical touch" for catheter guidance during embryo transfer in women. Cochrane Database Syst Rev. 2016;3:CD006107.
2. Porter MB. Ultrasound in assisted reproductive technology. Semin Reprod Med. 2008;26(3):266-76.
3. Henne MB, Milki AA. Uterine position at real embryo transfer compared with mock embryo transfer. Hum Reprod. 2004;19(3):570-2.
4. Woolcott R, Stanger J. Potentially important variables identified by transvaginal ultrasound-guided embryo transfer. Hum Reprod. 1997;12(5):963-6.
5. Gergely RZ, DeUgarte CM, Danzer H, Surrey M, Hill D, DeCherney AH. Three-dimensional/four-dimensional ultrasound-guided embryo transfer using the maximal implantation potential point. Fertil Steril. 2005;84(2):500-3.
6. Coroleu, B, Carreras O, Veiga A, Martell A, Martinez F, Belil I, et al. Embryo transfer under ultrasound guidance improves pregnancy rates after in-vitro fertilization. Hum Reprod. 2000;15:616-20.
7. Wood EG, Batzer FR, Go KJ, Gutmann JN, Corson SL. Ultrasound-guided soft catheter embryo transfers will improve pregnancy rates in in-vitro fertilization. Hum Reprod. 2000;15(1):107-12.

Normal and Abnormal Early Pregnancy

INTRODUCTION

A 12-week period immediately after fertilization of the ovum and formation of an embryo is the most eventful period of human life. A close observation of this period is a very useful guide to prognosis of pregnancy. Transvaginal scan is the modality of choice for documentation and assessment of early pregnancy. Volume ultrasound with transvaginal probe has brought a revolution in the study of embryology.

Before gestational sac appears: Blastocyst implants in the endometrium 5 days after fertilization of the ovum in the fallopian tube. One of the lips of endometrium in which implantation has occurred thickens and becomes hyperechoic due to the decidual reaction, and neoangiogenesis occurs to provide nutritional support to the embryo. Asymmetrical endometrial thickening **(Fig. 1A)** with low-resistance trophoblastic flow [resistance index (RI) <0.5 peak systolic velocity (PSV) >6 cm/s] in the thickened endometrial lip, points toward the implanting embryo. This is typically described as a "color comet sign"[1] **(Fig. 1B)**. With implantation, the progesterone secretion is enhanced from corpus luteum, and this is reflected as low-resistance blood flow to the corpus luteum (RI <0.5).

Scans are done during early pregnancy for:
- Confirmation of intrauterine pregnancy, its viability, and assessment of growth of pregnancy
- Diagnosing abnormal pregnancy
- Early detection of multiple gestations

CONFIRMATION OF INTRAUTERINE PREGNANCY

Beta-human chorionic gonadotropin (β-hCG) is the earliest and the first marker for confirmation of pregnancy, and gestational sac should be detected in the endometrial cavity on transvaginal scan when β-hCG levels are >1,000 IU/mL or as early as 4 weeks and 3–4 days from the 1st day of the last menstrual period and is diagnostic of intrauterine pregnancy.

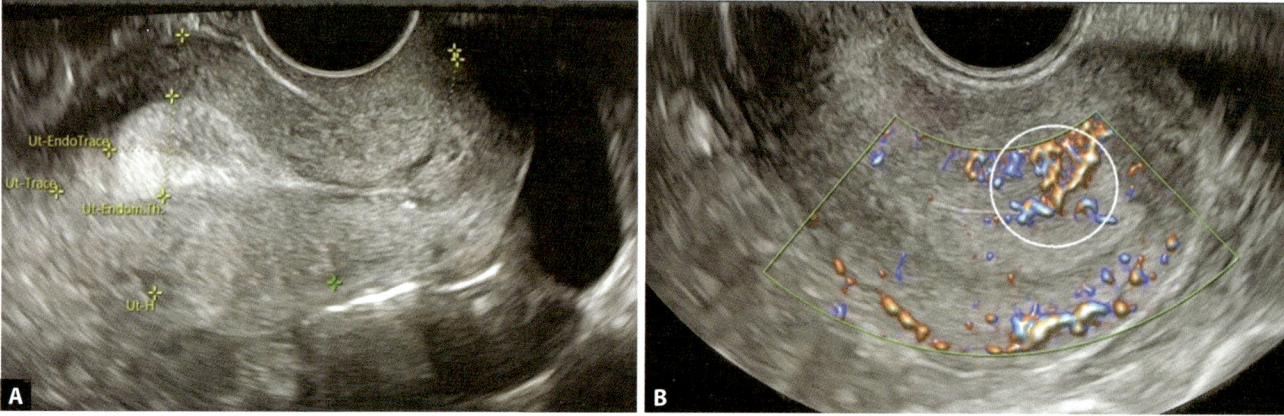

Figs. 1A and B: (A) Asymmetrical thickness of endometrial lips; (B) Color comet sign as shown in the white circle.

Normal and Abnormal Early Pregnancy

VIABILITY AND GROWTH OF THE PREGNANCY

The growth of the pregnancy occurs as described:

Four weeks: Gestational sac is a rounded anechoic structure, eccentrically placed in the endometrial cavity. It is 2–3 mm in diameter, with thick hyperechoic margins, due to decidual reaction—"double-decidual ring sign." On Doppler, it shows a ring of peripheral vascularity.

Five weeks: Yolk sac appears in the gestational sac as the first embryonic structure, at 5 weeks, 4 days. At the end of 5 weeks, the fetal pole of 1.5–2 mm is usually seen with cardiac activity seen in it as a flutter **(Fig. 2A)**.

Six weeks: Fetal pole elongates, caudal and cephalic poles can be identified, and crown-rump length reaches 4–8 mm in length. Omphalomesenteric duct is seen by the end of 6 weeks. Amniotic cavity is seen as a thin line surrounding the fetal pole by the end of 6th week **(Fig. 2B)**. It may appear similar to yolk sac in an image plane in which embryonic pole is not visible and is described as a "double-bleb sign".

Seven weeks: At this gestational age, the embryo may measure 9–14 mm. Rhombencephalon is seen in the cephalic end of the embryo. Umbilical cord is formed. Lower limb buds may be identified as tiny extensions toward the end of 7th week **(Fig. 2C)**.

Eight weeks: Head shows three brain vesicles, prosencephalon, mesencephalon, and rhombencephalon on sagittal section **(Fig. 2D)**. Development of the midline falx may become evident and choroid plexuses may be seen toward the end of the 8th week. The heart occupies about half of

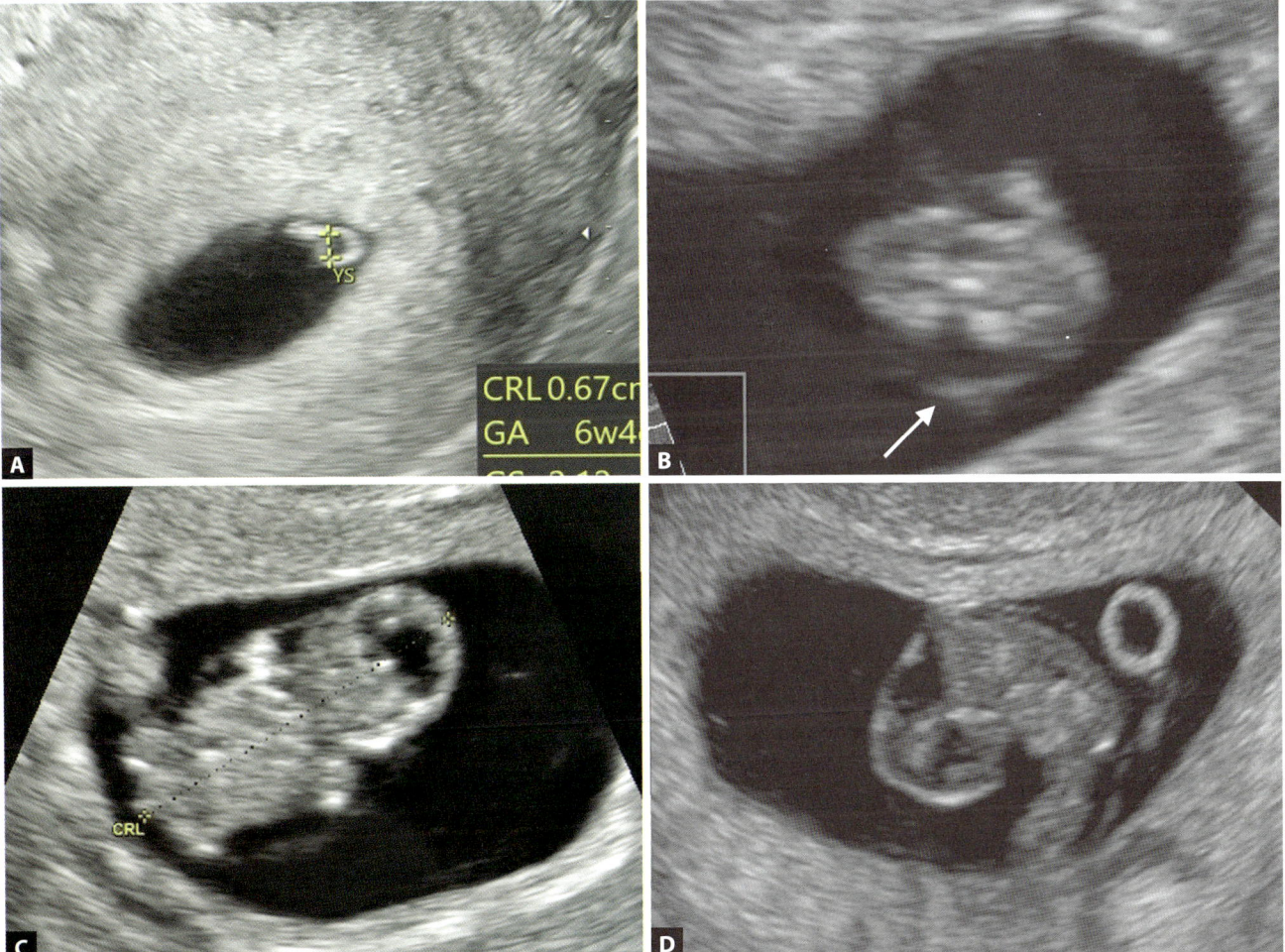

Figs. 2A to D: (A) 6 weeks pregnancy with yolk sac and embryonic pole; (B) 7 weeks gestation with elongated embryonic pole and amniotic sac (arrow); (C) Rhombencephalon and limb buds seen in the 7 weeks gestation; (D) Head shows three brain vesicles—prosencephalon, mesencephalon, and rhombencephalon on sagittal section, 8 weeks gestation.

the thoracic cavity. Atria and ventricle may be identifiable. Both upper and lower limb buds are seen. Physiological umbilical hernia is seen toward the end of the week. First fetal body movements also start around this time. Normal ultrasound at 8 weeks of pregnancy is a positive prognostic sign for a normal pregnancy outcome.

Nine weeks: Amniotic cavity occupies almost whole of gestational sac. The head appears larger than the body of the embryo. Elbows and knees are formed, and legs are bent medially to touch in midline. Limb movements can be appreciated. Falx is formed and choroid plexus fills up almost whole of the lateral ventricles. Spine starts forming and coccyx prominence can be identified. Orbital and oral pits start appearing. First, ossification centers of mandible and clavicle can be seen. Fetal circulation has already developed by this stage.

Ten weeks: Cerebellum is formed. Ossification of the skull starts from the occiput and at the end of first trimester, the skull thickness is 1 mm. Ossification of the spine starts. Fingers and toes are formed. Motion of atrioventricular valves and septa becomes visible in the heart. Omphalocele is largest at beginning of 10 weeks **(Fig. 3A)** and starts regressing at 10 weeks and 4 days. Circulation in aorta and carotids also may be seen.

Eleven weeks: Choroid plexus, falx, and calvarium are well formed **(Fig. 3B)**. Cerebral hemispheres start fusing in the midline. Cerebellum fuses in the midline. Spinal column can be seen. Heart is fully formed **(Fig. 3C)**. Stomach bubble becomes clear. Kidneys and urinary bladder can be seen. Omphalocele completely regresses at 11 weeks and 5 days.

Twelve weeks: Ossification of the spine progresses toward caudal end that had started at the cervical end. Each vertebra and intervertebral disk can be clearly identified. Metacarpals and metatarsals ossify. Kidneys, urinary bladder, and diaphragm can be identified at the start of 12th week in all fetuses. Facial details are clearly seen. Lens of the eye also can be identified.

■ ABNORMAL EARLY PREGNANCY

- Pregnancies with abnormal prognosis **(Flowchart 1)**
- Pregnancies of abnormal location **(Flowchart 2)**
- Pregnancies with uterine abnormalities
- Pregnancies with vesicular moles and chorioangiomas

An algorithmic approach to early pregnancy assessment is given in **Flowchart 1**.

Pregnancy with Abnormal Prognosis

- Abnormal growth pattern
- Anatomical/structural abnormalities
- *Fetal chromosomal abnormalities:* This is done on nuchal scan, after 11 weeks and requires a detailed assessment of the fetus and is out of the scope of this book.

Due to Abnormal Growth Pattern

Gestational sac, yolk sac, amniotic sac, and fetal pole all have a definite time of appearance and pace of growth.

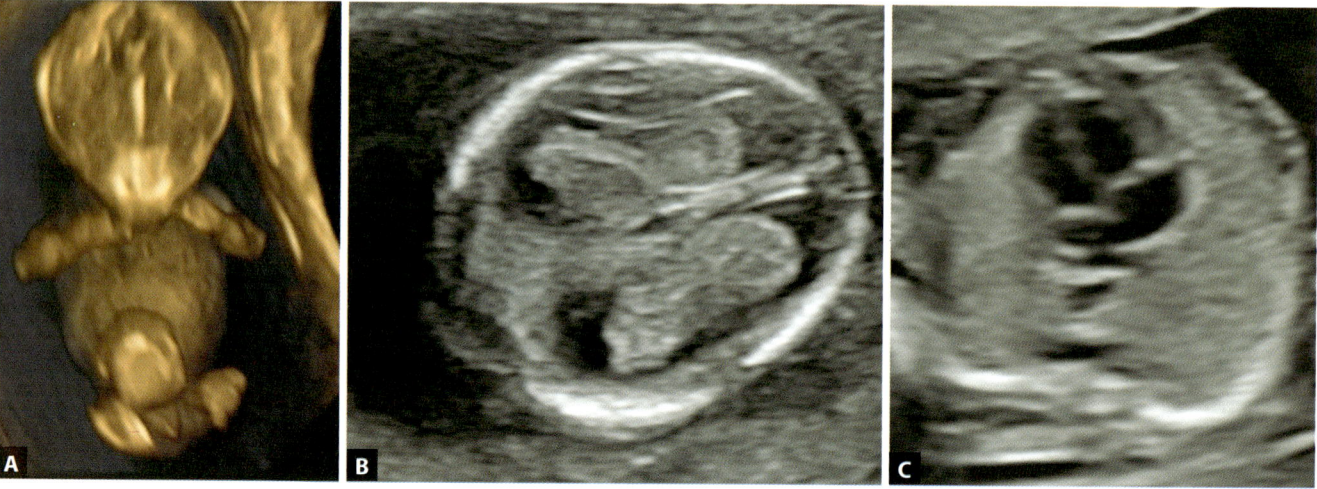

Figs. 3A to C: (A) 10 weeks fetus with omphalocele on 3D ultrasound; (B) 11 weeks fetal head with falx and choroid plexus; (C) 11 weeks fetal thorax with four chamber heart.

Normal and Abnormal Early Pregnancy

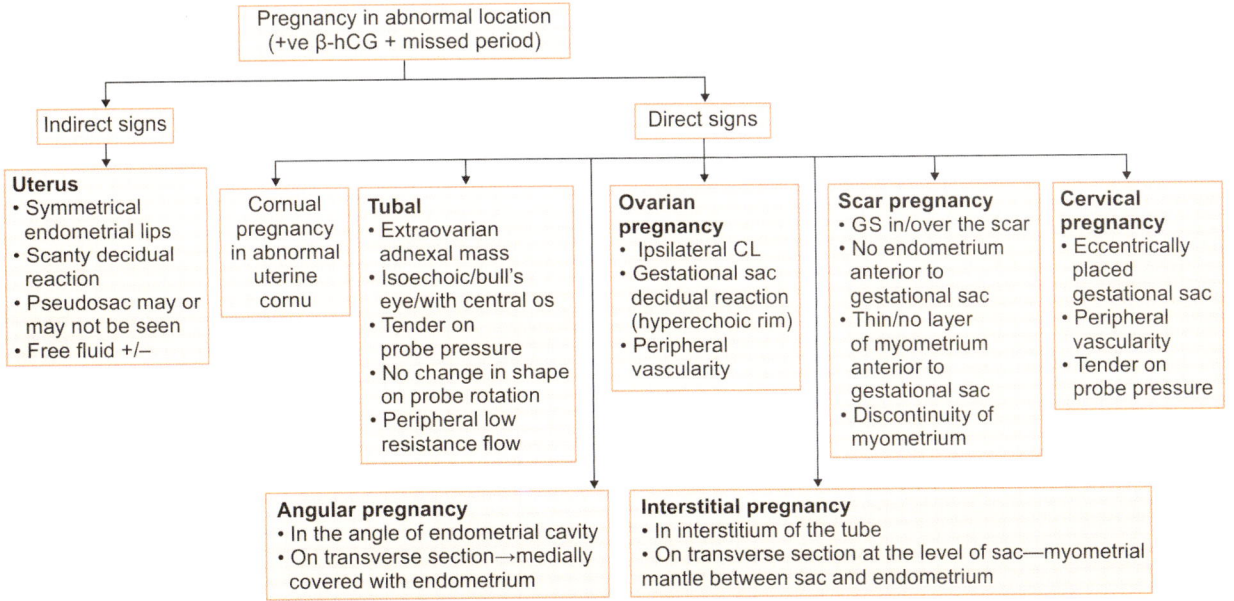

Flowchart 1: Early pregnancy assessment.

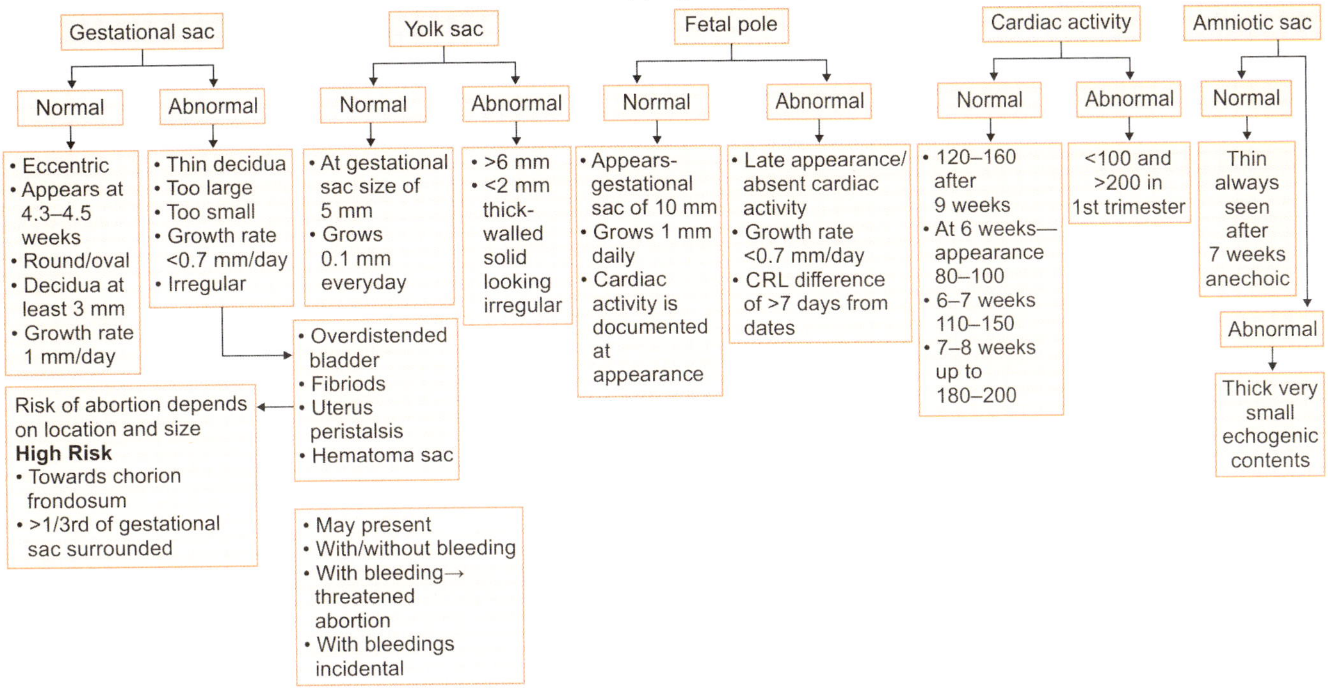

Flowchart 2: Pregnancies of abnormal location.

(CRL: crown-rump length; hCG: human chorionic gonadotropin)

These growth rates are very precise in first trimester and do not have genetic or individual variation. The technique for these measurements therefore should be standardized so that these parameters can assess the gestational age correctly and be used to detect any abnormality.

Gestational sac:
- Measured from inner edge to inner edge
- Always take a mean of three orthogonal diameters (orthogonal diameters are longest diameter on the long section of the gestational sac and the broadest

perpendicular to it and the third one is the longest side-to-side on the transverse section) **(Fig. 4A)**.
- Volume calculated by 3D ultrasound and virtual organ computer-aided analysis (VOCAL) software is now considered more reliable.

Abnormal gestational sac:
- Too large **(Fig. 4B)**
- Too small (abnormal size is to be diagnosed by plotting the measured values on the nomogram or growth charts) **(Fig. 4C)**.
- Does not have thick echogenic margins, decidual ring <3 mm. Trophoblastic thickness increases as pregnancy advances and is usually in first trimester ≥ the number of gestational weeks in millimeters.
- Appears late
- Absent or scanty vascularity, peripheral vascularity is considered abnormal.
- Yolk sac appears toward the end of the 4th week or when gestational sac is 10 mm in diameter. Fetal pole must be seen when gestational sac is 15 mm in diameter. If it does not, it may be a blighted ovum. But according to the guidelines, a gestational sac size of >20 mm with no yolk sac can be diagnosed as blighted ovum.[2]
- Irregular in shape **(Fig. 4D)**, this may be due to perisac hematoma, uterine contractions, fibroids, or overdistended bladder.
- Subchorionic hematomas **(Fig. 4E)** appear as anechoic area or an area with low-level echogenicity around the gestational sac. Though unobliterated endometrial cavity till about 8 weeks of gestation, it may also look similar.
- The location of the subchorionic hematoma can be correlated more with the risk of abortion than the size of the hematoma. A hematoma under the chorion frondosum indicates a poorer prognosis as compared to a hematoma under chorion leave and hematoma above the gestational sac have poorer prognosis than supracervical hematoma. A subchorionic hematoma that involves more than one-third of the gestational sac circumference also has a much higher risk of bad prognosis of pregnancy as compared to smaller hematomas.

Yolk sac **(Fig. 5A)**: It has nutritive, metabolic, endocrine, immunological, and hemopoietic functions. It must be seen after 7–8 days of visualization of the gestational sac.

Presence of yolk sac confirms embryonic pregnancy. It may start degenerating after 9 weeks but is often seen till end of 12 weeks.
- Measured inner wall to inner wall
- Grows 0.1 mm/day till 10 weeks, maximum 5–6 mm

Yolk sac is an indicator of poor outcome[3-5] if:
- Too small yolk sac <2 mm **(Fig. 5B)**
- Too large yolk sac >6 mm^2 **(Fig. 5C)**
- Thick-walled yolk sac **(Fig. 5D)**
- Solid yolk sac **(Fig. 5E)**
- Irregular yolk sac **(Fig. 5F)**

Fetal pole: It appears after the yolk sac. By transvaginal ultrasound, fetal cardiac activity can be detected at 5.6 weeks, approximately; when the fetal pole is approximately 1–2 mm in length. It is measured from the tip of the crown of the fetus to the tip of the rump, in a fetus in a neutral nonflexed, nonextended position that grows 1 mm/day. Size-to-date discrepancy of up to 5 days can be considered to be within normal limits. But when the difference in crown-rump length (CRL) is >7 mm of normal, it suggests higher risk of aneuploidy.

Amniotic membrane **(Fig. 6)**:
- Seen when CRL is 5–7 mm.
- 5.5 weeks—equal to yolk sac—double-bleb sign.
- Grows 1 mm/day.
- Fuses with chorion at about 14 weeks

Cardiac activity: It must always be seen at all times after 6 weeks of pregnancy.

Appearance of a fetal pole, without cardiac activity, is a sign of missed abortion.
- *Fifth week:* Slow like peristalsis; 60–80 beats/min
- *End of fifth week:* 100 beats/min
- *End of sixth week*: 105–130 beats/min
- *Nine weeks:* 160–170 beats/min, then 120–160 beats/min
- Heart rate of >200 beats/min is termed as tachycardia and <100 beats/min is termed as bradycardia in the first trimester.

Persistently, abnormal heart rate has a bad prognosis and late appearance of cardiac activity also indicates pregnancy with bad prognosis.

Fetal Abnormalities

Fetal abnormalities that can be detected in 1st trimester are as follows:

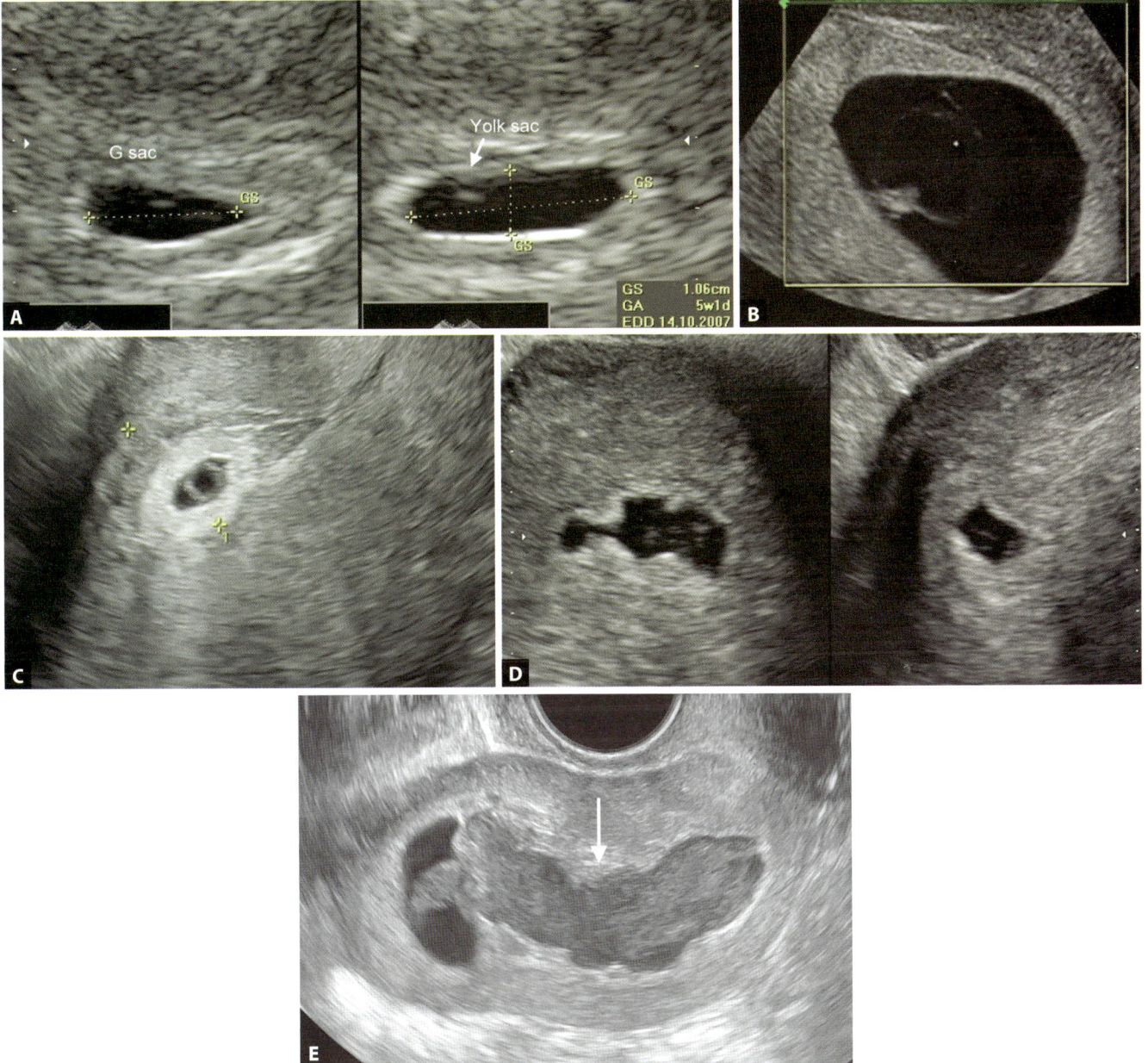

Figs. 4A to E: (A) Gestational sac seen in two orthogonal planes measured as three longest orthogonal diameters; (B) Large gestational sac; (C) Small gestational sac; (D) Irregular gestational sac; (E) Subchorionic hematoma (arrow). (G sac: gestational sac).

- *Acrania:* Acrania is lack of skull bone development. This leads to abnormal head shape as the developing brain tissue is directly exposed to amniotic fluid. The brain may appear echogenic and disorganized. This can be diagnosed as early as 9 weeks of gestation.
- *Holoprosencephaly (Fig. 7):* It is defect in division of prosencephalon due to defect in development of falx. If falx is not seen beyond 10th week, holoprosencephaly must be suspected. It may be seen in 24% of fetuses with trisomy 13.[6] Holoprosencephaly may vary in severity and may be classified as alobar, which is most severe with complete absence of falx, semilobar, and lobar. Alobar holoprosencephaly can always be diagnosed in the first trimester but lobar may be diagnosed beyond second trimester.
- *Major limb abnormalities:* All limb buds appear at 8 weeks and by the end of 10 weeks, all the segments of all 4 limbs are formed. Complete or partial absence

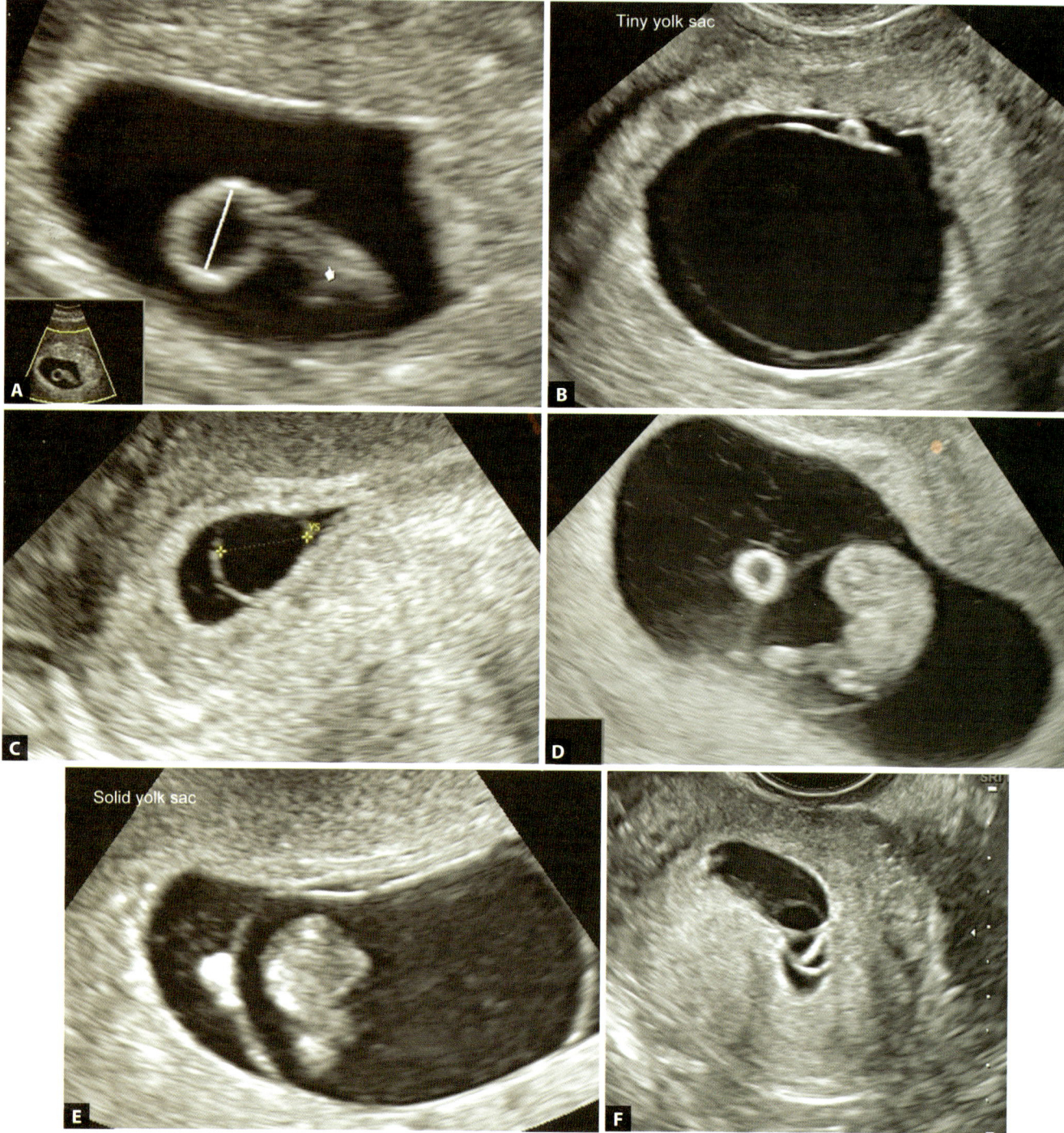

Figs. 5A to F: (A) Yolk sac measurement; (B) Tiny yolk sac; (C) Large yolk sac; (D) Thick-walled yolk sac; (E) solid yolk sac; (F) Irregular yolk sac.

of any of the limbs can be detected at all times after 10 weeks.
- *Major skeletal dysplasias* that can be diagnosed in first trimester include the following, but all are very rare.

- *Caudal regression syndrome (sirenomelia):* Absence of lower part of spine and fusion of lower limbs
- Body stalk abnormalities identified by anterior wall defect, kyphoscoliosis, limb reduction, and

Normal and Abnormal Early Pregnancy

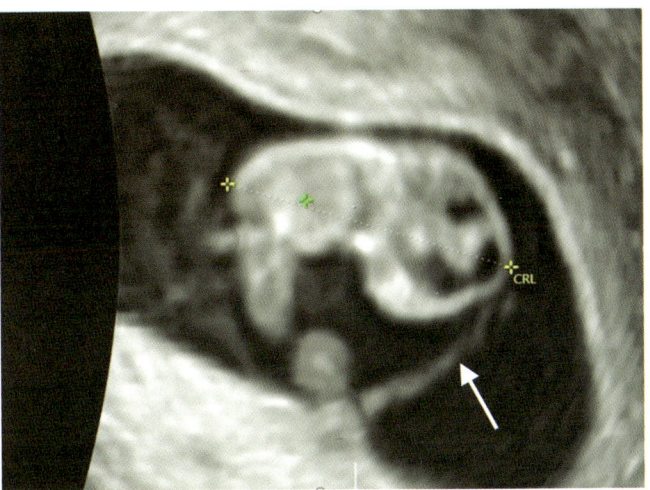

Fig. 6: 8–9 weeks pregnancy with amniotic sac (arrow).

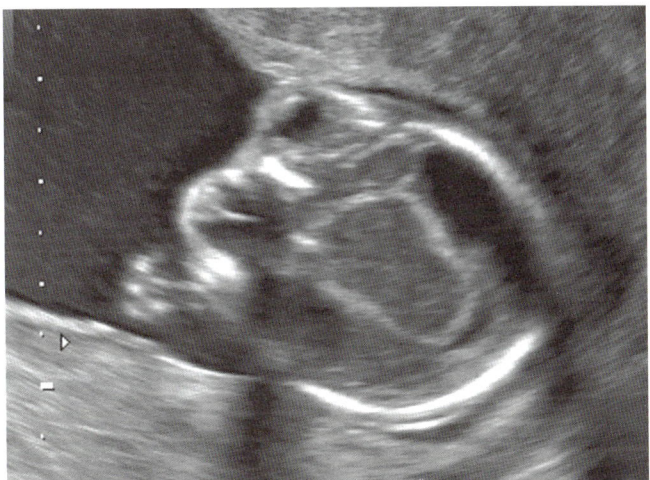

Fig. 7: Holoprosencephaly.

- *Major spinal defects:*
  - Open spina bifida can be diagnosed as early as 9 weeks, especially when associated with large meningocele or myelocele.[7]
  - Multiple vertebral abnormalities, hemivertebrae, etc. can also be diagnosed on first-trimester scans. Its prevalence is 1:1,000.
- *Abdominal wall defects:*
  - *Exomphalos (omphalocele):* This is a midline abdominal wall defect, through which abdominal viscera herniate out in a sac hernia. The umbilical cord is inserted at the apex of this sac. Omphalocele is physiological till 10 weeks of gestation, but if it persists after 11 weeks, it is pathological. Even before 10 weeks, if the neck of omphalocele is >7 mm or if on transverse section, the circumference of omphalocele is larger than the circumference of the fetal abdomen, it is pathological.
  - Gastroschisis is another anterior abdominal wall defect, usually on the right of the umbilical cord insertion. The bowel loops that herniate out of the abdominal cavity from this defect are floating free in amniotic fluid.
- *Abnormal location of gestational sac*—Ectopic gestation
  - Implantation of the gestational sac at any other location than endometrial cavity is considered abnormal and is termed as ectopic.
  - Patients with ectopic pregnancy typically present with a history of missed period with either fainting attacks, dizziness, or acute lower abdominal pain with raised β-hCG levels. The ultrasound diagnostic signs can be divided as uterine signs, extrauterine signs or indirect signs, and adnexal signs or direct signs. Uterine signs or indirect signs are similar in different locations of ectopic pregnancies, but the specific or direct signs are location-dependent.
- *Uterine signs:*
  - No intrauterine gestational sac with symmetrical endometrial lips **(Fig. 8A)**.
  - A pseudogestational sac may sometimes be seen in the uterus **(Fig. 8B)**

rudimentary umbilical cord, with body parts in celomic cavity.
- Achondrogenesis with severe shortening of limbs, narrow thorax, hypomineralization of vertebral bodies, but normal mineralization of skull
- Hypophosphatasia with hypomineralization of skull and spine, short ribs, and short long bones and Talipes equino varus (TEV).
- Osteogenesis imperfecta type II
- Short rib polydactyly syndrome
- *Major heart defects:* The cardiac abnormalities that can be diagnosed in first trimester are ectopia cordis, dextrocardia, monoventricular heart, atrioventricular septal defect, and major ventricular septal defect. Situs inversus can be always diagnosed in first trimester.

The psuedogestational sac can be differentiated from true sac by central location in endometrial cavity, absence of hyperechoic decidual rim, irregular shape, change in shape on peristalsis, and absence of vascularity.

Gestational sac at the lateral angles of the triangular endometrial cavity is known as angular pregnancy

(Figs. 8C and D). Majority of these pregnancies grow medially toward the endometrial cavity and may not have any negative consequences further in pregnancy, except a risk of abnormally adherent placenta. Gestational sac in the interstitium of the fallopian tube (interstitial pregnancy) **(Figs. 8E and F)** usually cannot grow beyond 8 weeks and can lead to serious complications. This is because the interstitial part of the tube is covered by myometrium. Correct and timely diagnosis of this is important. On transverse section of fundus of the uterus, gestational sac is seen lateral to the lateral edge of the uterine cavity and is surrounded only by a thin layer of myometrium; this is interstitial pregnancy. Whereas in angular pregnancy, medially the sac is in continuity with the endometrium, but lateral to the gestational sac, no endometrial mantle is seen.

Cornual pregnancy is a gestational sac that is implanted in one of the cornua of congenitally abnormal uterus **(Fig. 8G)**.

Gestational sac may also be implanted in the cervix and is known as cervical pregnancy **(Fig. 8F)** and is typically seen as ballooning of the cervix and hourglass shape of the uterus. Cervical pregnancy can be differentiated from gestational sac in process of abortion by the surrounding vascularity, eccentric location, and regular shape of the gestational sac in cervical pregnancy compared to no vascularity, irregular shape, and central location for the gestational sac which is in process of abortion.

Rarely gestational sac may implant in a uterine scar of previous surgery also.

Scar pregnancy **(Fig. 8H)** includes pregnancy in the scar and pregnancy over the scar. It is the pregnancy in the scar that is more dangerous. This leads to opening of the scar and uterine rupture. Whereas pregnancy over the scar is a gestational sac that is implanted on the scar but then grows in the endometrial cavity, these pregnancies have a high risk of pathologically adherent placenta.

The most common location for extrauterine ectopic pregnancy is the fallopian tube but may be seen in the ovary or free in the peritoneal cavity.

Adnexal Signs

Any adnexal mass in a female with a missed period and positive blood or urine pregnancy test is considered to be ectopic pregnancy unless proved otherwise. It may be with or without true gestational sac. The mass is typically described to have a central anechoic area with surrounding hyperechoic rim of decidual reaction surrounded by a thick isoechoic wall and a peripheral rim of vascularity with low resistance flow **(Figs. 9A and B)**. But it is important to remember that this typical appearance develops late during the development of ectopic tubal pregnancy. The earliest ultrasound sign will be an extraovarian isoechoic lesion in the adnexa with peripheral vascularity, which is tender on probe pressure.

Ipsilateral active corpus luteum and free fluid in pelvis are additional ultrasound signs. Early diagnosis of ectopic pregnancy helps conservative management and decreases morbidity.

Ovarian ectopic: It is anechoic circular gestational sac in ovary with typical hyperechoic decidual reaction like rim, with peripheral vascularity. This can be differentiated from a corpus luteum only by its hyperechoic rim **(Fig. 9C)**.

Abdominal ectopic pregnancy: Abdominal/peritoneal ectopic gestational sac is seen lying free outside uterus, tubes or ovaries. It is usually surrounded by fluid. It is very difficult to locate as it can be placed anywhere in the peritoneal cavity.

And when not being able to locate it, it is diagnosed as pregnancy of unknown origin. Then it is followed up by beta-hCG levels to decide the further line of treatment.

PREGNANCY WITH UTERINE ABNORMALITIES

Uterine abnormalities are likely to lead to poor prognosis of pregnancy. Fibroids when submucosal are likely to lead to implantation failures and early abortions due to distortion of endometrial cavity. Larger fibroids may interfere with the circulation to the endometrium and also hamper normal peristalsis and therefore may lead to pregnancy failures. Apart from pregnancy failure, fibroids may lead to severe pain due to degenerative changes and enlargement of the fibroid. Moreover, fibroids are also likely to enlarge and cause severe pain during pregnancy. Fibroids may also lead to bleeding during early pregnancy.

This is due to hypercirculatory pregnancy state. Saravelos et al.[7] have shown in their study that myomas are more commonly associated with midtrimester losses and resecting the fibroids that distort the endometrial cavity can double the live birth rate in subsequent pregnancies. Adenomyosis also is known to lead to early abortion and early pregnancy bleeding.

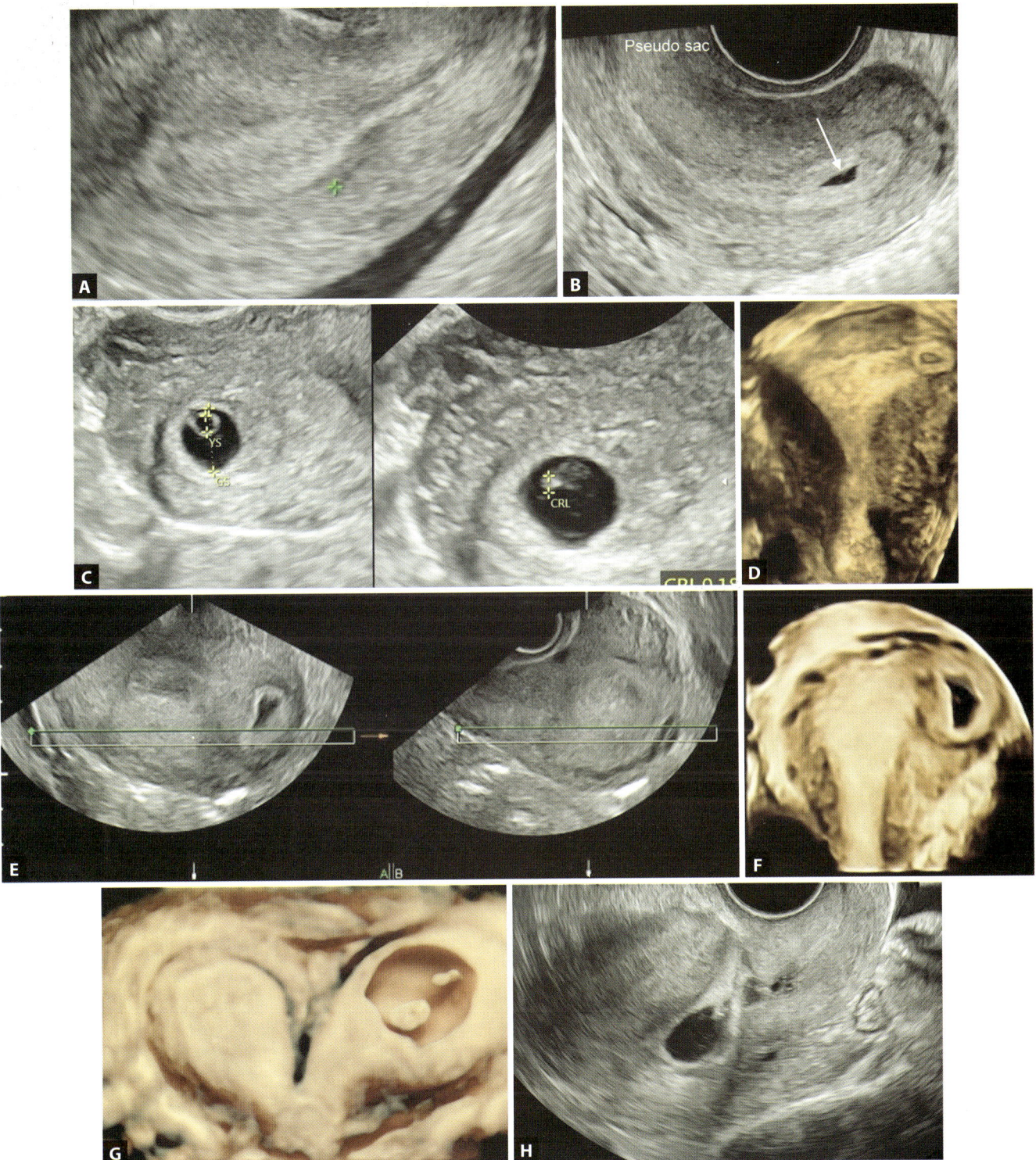

Figs. 8A to H: (A) Symmetrical endometrial lips indicating that gestational sac is not implanted in the endometrial cavity; (B) Pseudogestational sac (arrow); (C) B-mode image; (D) 3D ultrasound image with angular pregnancy; (E) B-mode ultrasound; (F) 3D ultrasound image of interstitial pregnancy; (G) Cornual pregnancy in the left horn of bicornuate uterus; (H) Pregnancy in the cesarean scar.

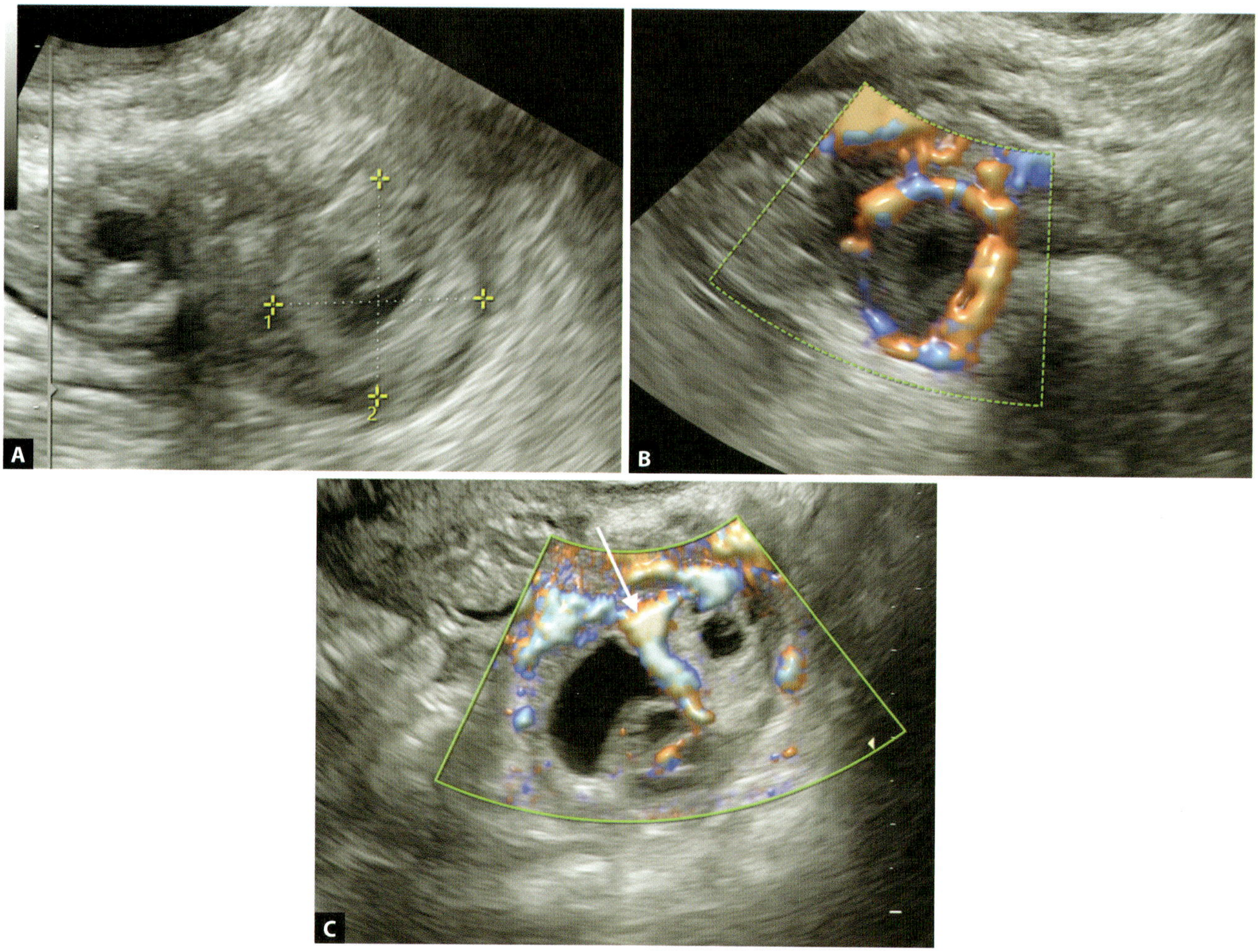

Figs. 9A to C: (A) B-mode and (B) HD flow Doppler image of ectopic pregnancy; (C) Ovarian ectopic pregnancy with peripheral vascularity (arrow).

PREGNANCIES WITH TUMORS OF CHORIONIC TISSUE

Chorioangioma **(Fig. 10):** Chorioangiomas can be seen in early pregnancy (7–8 weeks of pregnancy) as solid isoechoic tissue balls. Small chorioangiomas do not affect the pregnancy, but larger ones may lead to circulatory failures in fetus due to circulatory overload.

Vesicular mole **(Figs. 11A and B):** High β-hCG levels with absent gestational sac with thick echogenic endometrium that has small anechoic areas are diagnostic of vesicular mole. In early phases, vascularity may not be picked up on Doppler studies due to low-velocity flow. Only when it becomes invasive, it disrupts the endometrial–myometrial junction and then is usually large enough to show abundant low-resistance vascularity.

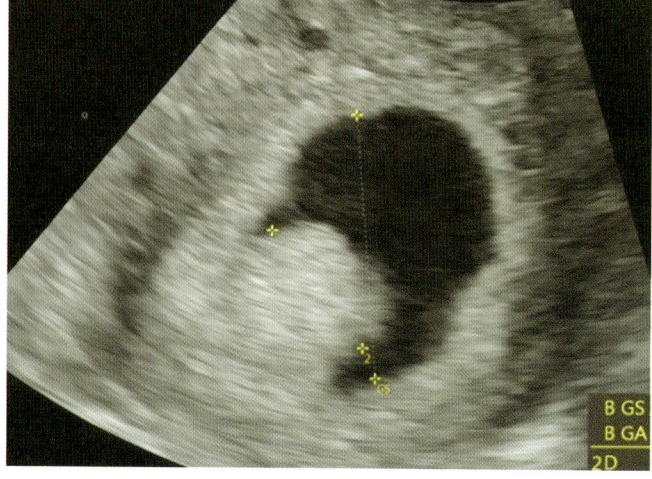

Fig. 10: B-mode image of chorioangioma.

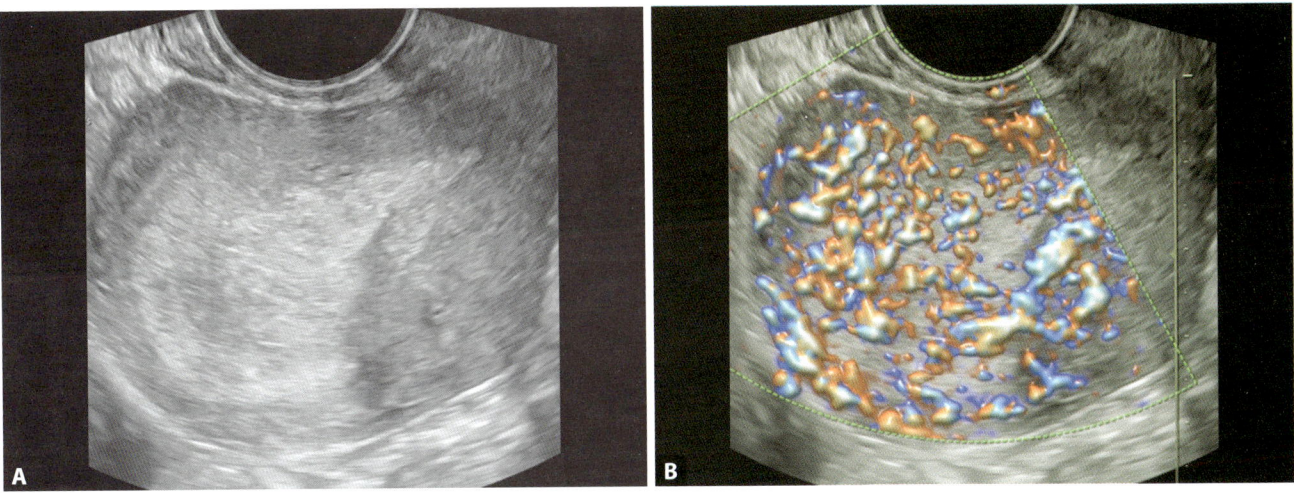

Figs. 11A and B: (A) B-mode; (B) HD flow image of vesicular mole.

Early detection of multiple gestations: Multiple gestations have much higher complication rates than singleton pregnancy. The complication rate and management are different for monochorionic and dichorionic and monoamniotic and diamniotic pregnancies. It is, therefore, essential to confirm the chorionicity and amnionicity of any multiple gestations. This can be best done at 6–8 weeks of pregnancy. This is the time when gestational sacs are small and, therefore, individual sac margins can be confidently identified. This may be done in later pregnancy by lambda sign. But this may also become less obvious in the late second trimester.

CONCLUSION

- Assessment of early pregnancy is of utmost importance.
- Ultrasound is the tool of choice.
- Route of the scan should always be transvaginal.
- Bleeding during pregnancy is not a contraindication to assessment by vaginal route.

REFERENCES

1. Honemeyer U, Kurjak A, Monni G. Normal and abnormal early pregnancy. In: Kurjak A, Chervenak F (Eds). Donald School Textbook of Ultrasound in Obstetrics and Gynecology, 2nd edition. New Delhi: Jaypee Brothers Medical Publishers 2008. pp. 106-29.
2. Jeve Y, Rana B, Bhide A, Thangaratinam S. Accuracy of first trimester ultrasound in the diagnosis of early embryonic demise: a systematic review. Ultrasound Obstet Gynecol. 2011;38(5):489-96.
3. Lyons EA. Endovaginal sonography of the first trimester of pregnancy. Proceedings of the third International Perinatal and Gynecological Ultrasound Symposium, Ottawa, Ontario. 1994. pp. 1-25.
4. Bromley B, Harlow BL, Laboda LA, Benacerraf BR. Small sac size in the first trimester: a predictor for poor fetal outcome. Radiology. 1991;178(2):375-7.311
5. Green JJ, Hobbins JC. Abdominal ultrasound examination of the first trimester fetus. Am J Obstet Gynecol. 1988;159(1):165-75.
6. Blass HG, Eik-Nes SH, Isaksen CV. The detection of spina bifida before 10 gestational weeks using two- and three-dimensional ultrasound. Ultrasound Obstet Gynecol. 2000;16(1):25-9.
7. Saravelos SH, Yan J, Rehmani H, Li TC. The prevalence and impact of fibroids and their treatment on the outcome of pregnancy in women with recurrent miscarriage. Hum Reprod. 2011;26(12):3274-9.

Anatomy of Pelvic Floor and Diagnosis of Descents

INTRODUCTION

Urogynecology deals with the assessment of the pelvic floor and diagnosis of pathologies caused by its abnormalities. The most common cause for urogynecological abnormalities is pelvic floor trauma during labor. About 10–30% of all women having delivered vaginally have some avulsion of puborectalis. Over 40% of women undergoing normal labor suffer either Frank tears or irreversible overdistention of hiatus.[1]

Common complaints are recurrent urinary tract infection, persistent dysuria, urgency, frequency, urinary incontinence, genitourinary prolapse, flatus, and fecal incontinence. These more commonly affect postmenopausal females, but symptoms are not uncommon in premenopausal women too. The real incidence is difficult to document because even though its awareness and therefore seeking medical help for the same is increasing in developed countries, but in many more countries, there is still a hesitation to complain and present for the same.

COMPLAINTS AND CLINICAL HISTORY

Complaints and clinical history often help to direct to the correct diagnosis, especially in cases of stress urinary incontinence. Important points in history are duration and the severity of incontinence and differentiation between incontinence, urgency, and difficulty in voiding. Detailed clinical history, actually, in these cases is half the diagnosis.

PHYSICAL EXAMINATION

Physical examination chiefly includes assessing for vulvovaginitis, atrophic changes, prolapse of bladder, bowel, or vault, and presence of pelvic masses. Neurological disease may often be the basis for the complaints. Patients with incontinence and prolapse must be assessed also with coughing or Valsalva. Tone of the pelvic floor muscles is assessed with at least digital palpation.

INVESTIGATIONS

Investigations include (**Flowchart 1**):
- Urine analysis
- *Transabdominal ultrasound:* For kidneys, ureters, and bladder
- *Transvaginal ultrasound:* For uterus, adnexa, and ovaries
- *Transperineal ultrasound:* For assessment of the pelvic floor. B-mode ultrasound allows us to evaluate the internal pelvic anatomy, but not the pelvic floor muscles as these are perpendicular to the probe surface (**Figs. 1A and B**).
- *Three-dimensional (3D)–4D transperineal ultrasound:* 3D pelvic floor ultrasound enables us to evaluate the levator ani and is both operator and patient-friendly (**Fig. 2**).[2,3]

Rendered image or omniview with volume contrast imaging (VCI) on 3D ultrasound can also be used to assess the pelvic floor muscles.[4] At least three central slices taken of omniview are used; plane of minimum hiatal dimensions and two slices 2.5 and 5 mm cranial to it. Lower most slice is just below the insertion of puborectalis muscle.[5] Tomographic ultrasound imaging may also be a valuable and time saving option.

Levator hiatus is space between these various muscles and through that, the orifices, urethra, vagina, and anus are seen.[6] Puborectalis, extend from public symphysis till behind the anus.[7] The latter is the most important muscle to maintain continence and control. 3D/4D transperineal ultrasound (TUS) can identify specific avulsion of puborectalis muscle. It is the result of the detachment of the muscle from its insertion on the inferior pubic ramus

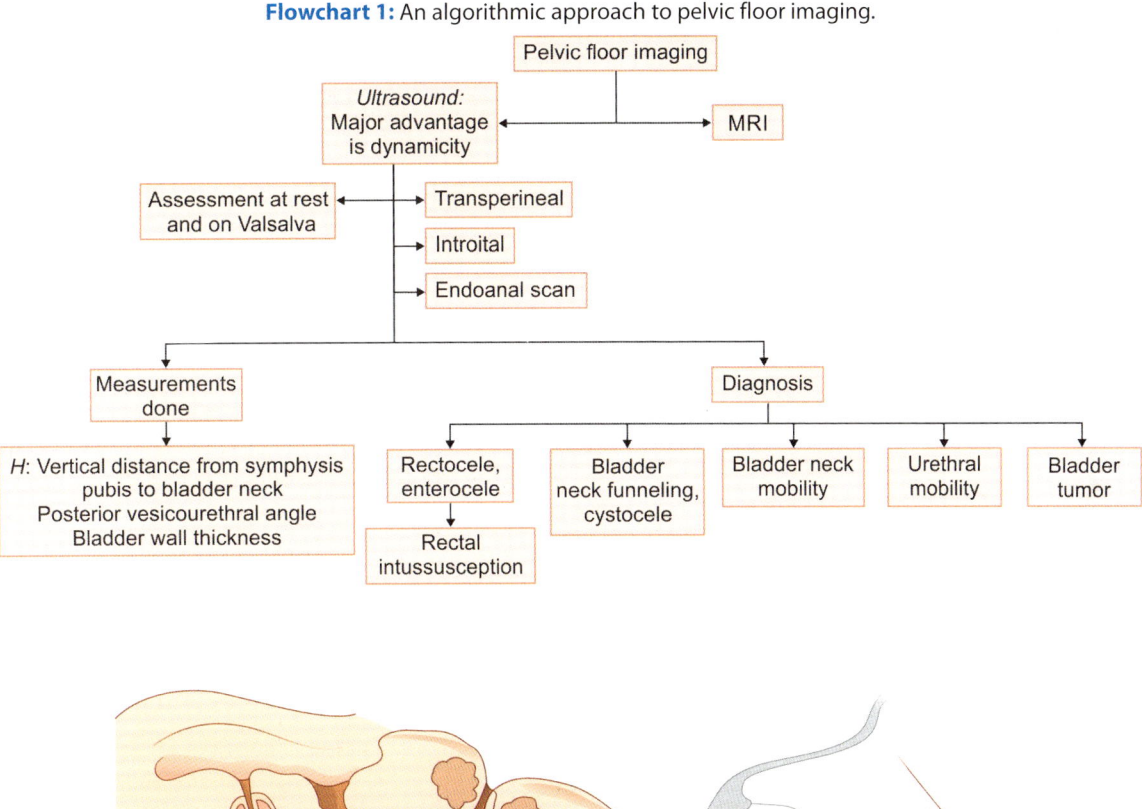

Flowchart 1: An algorithmic approach to pelvic floor imaging.

Figs. 1A and B: (A) A anatomical diagram of the basic anatomy of the prineal region; (B) Diagrammatic representation of the anatomy of female pelvis as seen on transperineal scan. (S: symphysis pubis, U: uterus; US: ultrasound probe)

as a consequence of overstretching of the levator during the second stage of labor and may be detected in up to 36% of women following their first vaginal delivery.

Transperineal Ultrasound

Transperineal ultrasound is carried out with a 3.5–6 MHz curved array transducer placed on the perineum in the midsagittal line. Transducer is covered with glove. Examination is usually performed in the dorsal lithotomy position with the hips flexed and abducted. For perineal ultrasound, probe is placed over the labia. Parting of labia may be required for better image quality. Transducer is placed firmly on symphysis pubis (SP) and perineum. Acquisition angle should be of 80° or more to include the entire pelvis. One volume is acquired at rest and one on Valsalva.

The resulting image contains the SP, urethra, bladder, vagina, rectum, and anal canal **(Figs. 3A to C)**. The SP

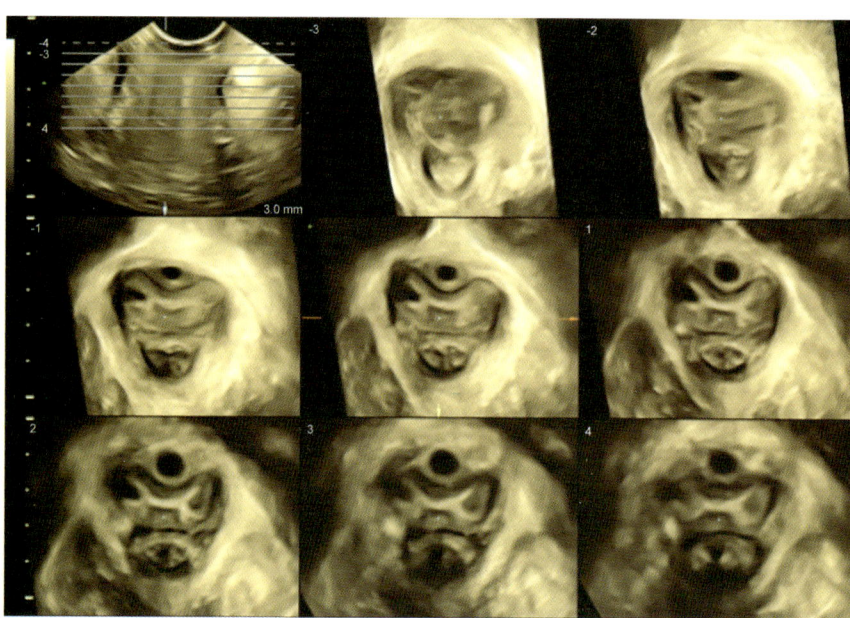

Fig. 2: 3D ultrasound with tomographic ultrasound imaging of the pelvic floor, showing axial sections of perineum at different levels.

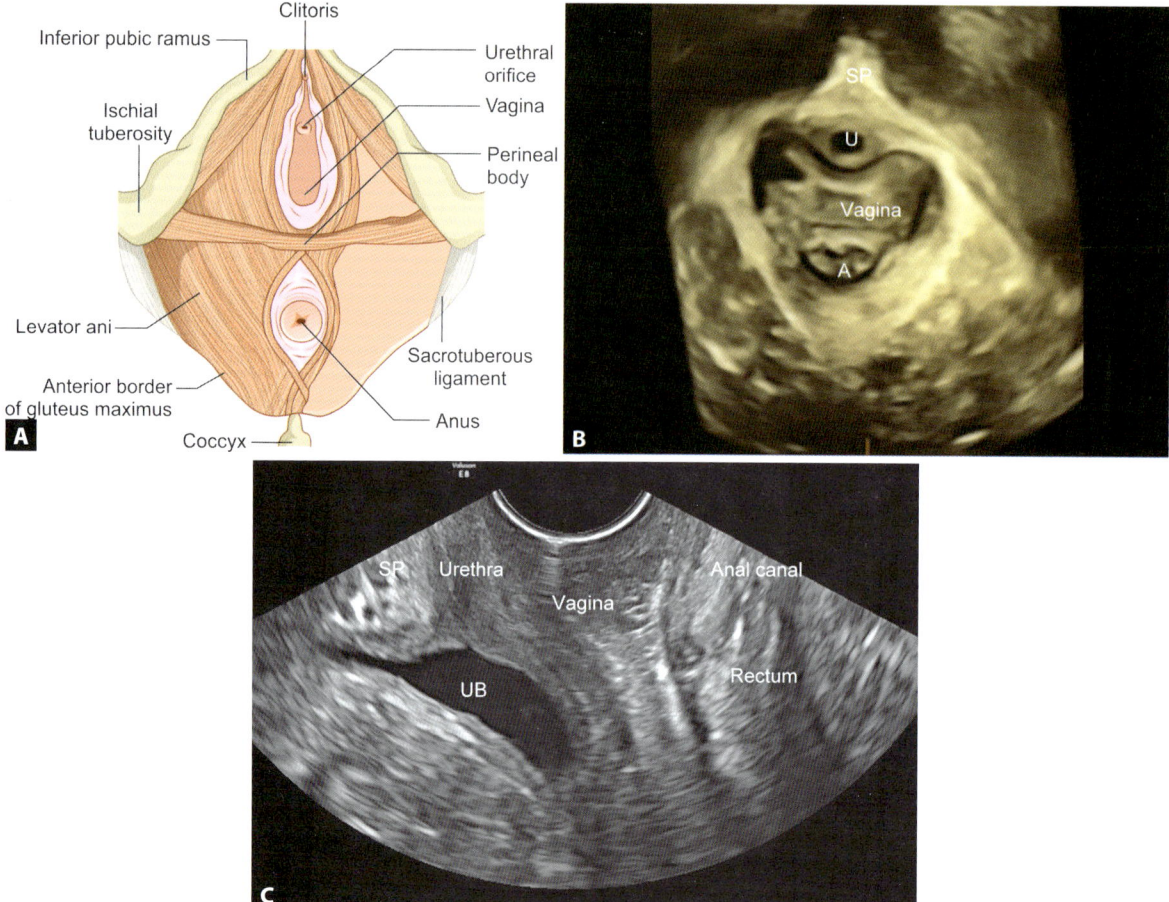

Figs. 3A to C: (A and B) Diagrammatic anatomical section and 3D ultrasound axial section of the pelvic floor; (C) Midsagittal section of the pelvic floor, depicting the anatomy. (A: Anus; SP: symphysis pubis; U: urethra)

is used as a stable landmark serving as a reference for evaluation of the bladder neck position and mobility.

Since the technique enables one to obtain tomographic or multislice scans, the whole puborectalis muscle and its attachments to the pubic rami can be visualized.[3,8,9]

Introital Ultrasound

The technique involves the use of front-firing endovaginal probes (5–7.5 MHz) placed on the vaginal introitus. It provides higher resolution of images but has reduced penetration into the tissues. The effect of the Valsalva maneuver on proximal urethra mobility may be evaluated along with TUS using the inferior margin of the SP as a reference.[10,11] For introital scan, the probe is placed over external urethral orifice, with long axis of the probe along the long axis of the body. This scan shows only lower end of SP. Primarily assessment of the urethra, urinary bladder, periurethral tissues, endopelvic fascia, vagina, and rectum is done. Excessive pressure is never exerted on the probe. This may displace the bladder neck. The assessment is done at rest, on coughing, on Valsalva, and with pressure.

Measurements routinely taken are as follows:
- *H:* Vertical distance between lower end of SP to the bladder neck (20.6 mm at rest and 14 mm on pressing).[12-14]
- *Angle B:* Posterior urethrovesical angle is between long axis of urethra and bladder neck. Assessment is done at rest, during contraction, coughing, and pressing[15] (normal at rest = 96.8° and on pressure = 108.1).[12-14]
- *Bladder wall thickness (BWT):* Best measured after micturition in lithotomy position, on transvaginal scan.[16] Measurement is done at the thickest part of the trigone dome and anterior wall of urinary bladder.
- *Bladder neck funneling:* This is not seen at rest. But if incontinence is present, funneling must be seen, unless examination is done in lying down position, with empty bladder, or with inadequate Valsalva pressure.[17]
- *Bladder neck mobility:* It may be influenced by pregnancy and delivery apart from body habitus. Mobility can decrease with pelvic floor awareness education.[18,19] Rotational posteroinferior descent with inferior margin of symphysis acting as a pivot documents bladder neck hypermobility.

Some workers also assess the levator ani thickness.

Maximum levator thickness is determined by slowly moving the plane of minimal hiatal dimensions cranially until the plane of maximal thickness of the pubovisceral muscle is reached. This is usually located about 1–1.5 cm above the actual levator hiatus. Though the thickness of muscle mass did not correlate with levator function, a bulky levator may not necessarily contract well.[20]

In the axial view, maximum diameters of the pubovisceral muscle in two locations bilaterally and muscle area by tracing its outline at the level of maximal muscle thickness can also be assessed. It leads to enlargement of the levator hiatus, which on 4D TUS is observed as a "hiatus ballooning". Both levator avulsion and ballooning are associated with pelvic organ prolapse (POP).[3,8,9]

Endoanal Route

Endoanal route is selected for anal incontinence and anal tumors. It can also be used for assessment of anal sphincter. Ultrasound is an optional test in the evaluation of patients with complex or recurrent urinary incontinence (UI) and/or (POP) (Level of evidence 3, Grade of recommendation C).

■ B-MODE ULTRASOUND

B-mode ultrasound is done to look for:
- Bladder volume
- BWT
- Bladder tumors
- Urethral diverticula (UD)
- Hematomas
- Bladder neck mobility
- Cystocele/Cystourethrocele
- Enterocele/Rectocele
- Rectal intussusception (RI)

Bladder Volume Measurement (Fig. 4)

Bladder volume measurement is especially done in cases of:
- Overactive bladder syndrome
- Neurogenic bladder
- Pelvic prolapse
- Voiding symptoms
- After incontinence surgeries

It is always done on transabdominal scan.

The recent International Federation of Gynecology and Obstetrics (FIGO) Group guidelines, in concert with other recommendations, advise that postvoid volumes greater than 150 mL should be regarded as abnormal.[21]

Higher incidence of elevated postvoid residual (PVR) is observed among patients with stress urinary incontinence (SUI), previous incontinence surgery, overactive bladder,

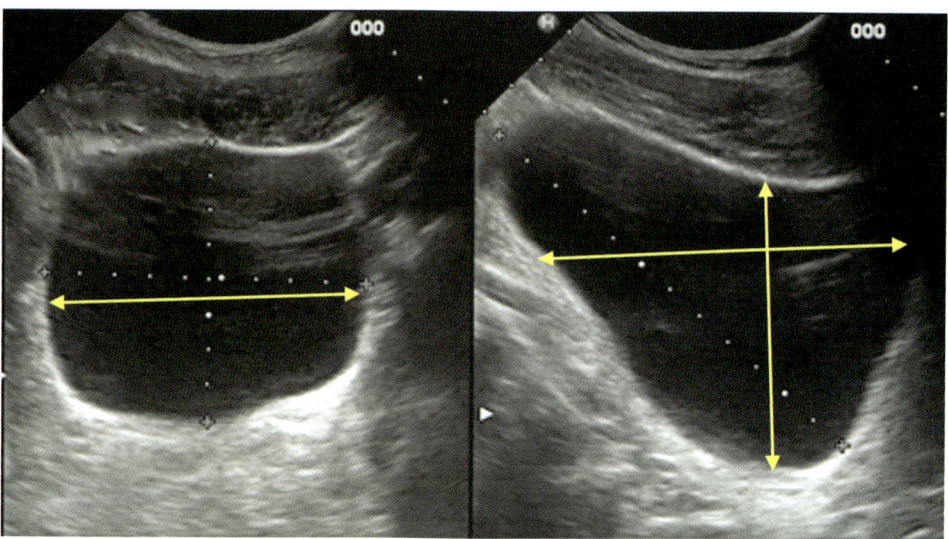

Fig. 4: Transabdominal B-mode ultrasound scan of transverse and long axis of urinary bladder with 3 longest orthogonal diameter measurement.

multiple sclerosis, and POP stage 2 or greater.[21] According to Tseng et al., almost 16% of women with SUI have PVR >100 mL.[22]

Ultrasound estimations may be performed using either three diameters (length, height, and width) or the surface area in the transverse image and the length obtained in the longitudinal image.

Bladder Wall Thickness as a Marker of Detrusor Overactivity

Increased BWT or detrusor wall thickness (DWT) is seen in patients with detrusor overactivity (DO). Using a 5-mm cut-off for BWT for identifying DO, the sensitivity and specificity of this marker were 85% and 89% in one study[13] but 40% and 79% in another.[23] BWT is measured at three places: Anterior wall, trigone, and the dome and a mean value is taken. Though there are insufficient data to reliably estimate accuracy of BWT in DO. BWT is also seen with infection after radiation or surgery, in neurological bladder, detrusor instability, outflow tract obstruction, and neoplasm.

Bladder Tumors

Bladder tumors are polypoid/sessile solid projections or plaque-like with regular or irregular surfaces and with or without calcifications. Bladder wall invasion is checked by sliding organ sign.[24] Bladder endometriotic nodule may also look very similar to plaque-like tumor growth **(Figs. 5A and B)**.

Urethral Diverticula

Urethral diverticula may be observed in up to 1.4% of those with urinary incontinence.[25-27] The classic presentation of UD includes dysuria, dyspareunia, and (post-void) dribbling, but may also present with frequency, urgency, UI, pain, or discharge. Most probably, UD is a consequence of chronic inflammation.[28] The majority of diverticula appear like a simple pouch, but some can have complex morphology such as saddlebag or circumferential. On transvaginal ultrasound these are seen as cystic lesions (single/multiple) around the urethra.[29]

Retropubic Hematoma

Retropubic hematoma is seen following retropubic urethropexy or suburethral sling procedure. On transvaginal scan, it appears as hypoechoic or mixed echogenic area between SP, urethra, and bladder.

Bladder neck funneling (opening of the bladder neck on Valsalva or coughing) is a typical finding in women with SUI but can be seen in asymptomatic women as well.[13,30,31]

Urethral Hypermobility (Bladder Neck Mobility)

On transperineal or introital ultrasound, the position of the bladder neck at rest and on maximal Valsalva may be determined relative to the inferoposterior margin of the

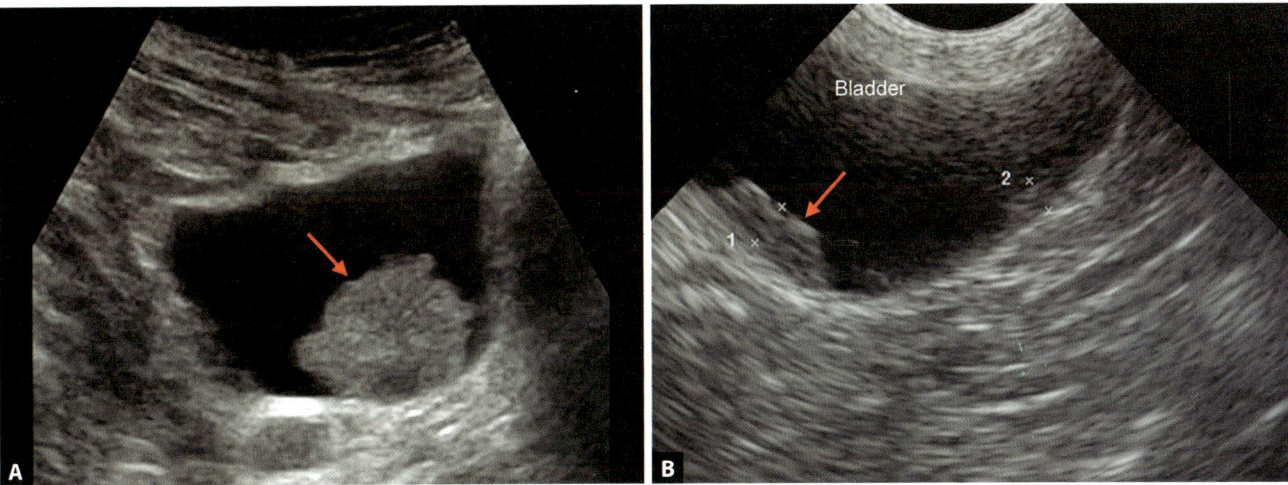

Figs. 5A and B: (A) B-mode ultrasound image of urinary bladder with solid projection—neoplasm seeen in the bladder; (B) B-mode ultrasound image of the urinary bladder with a plaque-like solid projection seen between 6 and 9 o'clock position (arrow).

SP. On Valsalva, the bladder neck and proximal urethra rotate in the posteroinferior direction. This results in an urge to pass urine immediately after voiding once or as stress incontinence. Valsalva maneuver is forced expiration against closed glottis, contracted diaphragm, and abdominal wall and must be continued for at least 5 seconds. It is important that the maneuver is properly explained to the patient and rehearsed because most of the time when patient is asked to exert pressure in downward direction, like in Valsalva, she actually uplifts the pelvic floor and holds it tight. This is called levator coactivation. This may mask both the hypermobility of bladder neck as well as the prolapse. Levator coactivation can be differentiated from the Valsalva on imaging by assessing the reduced anteroposterior diameter of levator hiatus with elevation of anorectum **(Figs. 6A to D)** and increase in anteroposterior diameter of the levator hiatus with downward movement of anorectum suggests Valsalva **(Figs. 7A to C)**.

Measurements are taken at rest and on maximal straining. The hypermobility of the urethra is not well defined, and different cutoffs of 20, 25, or 30 mm have been proposed.[10,32] Though in one study, among nulliparous continent women of approximately 20 years of age, the bladder neck descent varied between 1 mm and 40 mm.[33]

Endopelvic fascia and anterior vaginal wall form a supportive layer on which urethra courses.[34,35] Reactivity of the pelvic floor can be assessed by measuring the distance from lower margin of pubic symphysis to bladder neck (H). Increased distance reflects good levator ani reactivity.[36]

Cystocele

With hypermobility of the urethra, there may also be hypermobility of the bladder. This allows a pouch of the bladder to descend below the level of the bladder neck and this results in urinary retention. This urine-filled pocket of bladder protrudes on the anterior vaginal wall as cystocele. Vertical descent of the urethra may also be associated with descent of bladder and cystocele. Ultrasound imaging enables one to discriminate between cystourethrocele and isolated cystocele in the anterior compartment, and between rectocele and enterocele in the posterior compartment.[17]

Transperineal ultrasound can be used to quantify the degree of prolapse. A fairly good correlation between ultrasound and clinical prolapse assessment has been demonstrated.

Vaginal wall or vault prolapse: Defined as descent of anterior urethrovesical junction or any point on the anterior vaginal wall <3 cm from the hymenal ring.[37] Low uterus may compress posteriorly and obscure rectocele. Retroverted uterus with uterine descent may lead to voiding dysfunction. For the prolapse or descent, it has been shown that the levator hiatal size at rest closely correlates with the possibility of descent even in absence of trauma.[38] The hiatal size is measured as shown in the **Figure 8**. Hiatal overdistention may be present due to microtrauma, even in absence of avulsion **(Figs. 9A and B)**. It is diagnosed by increase in more than 20% hiatal area (hiatus >25 cm^2). 25 cm^2 is the upper limit of normal hiatus.

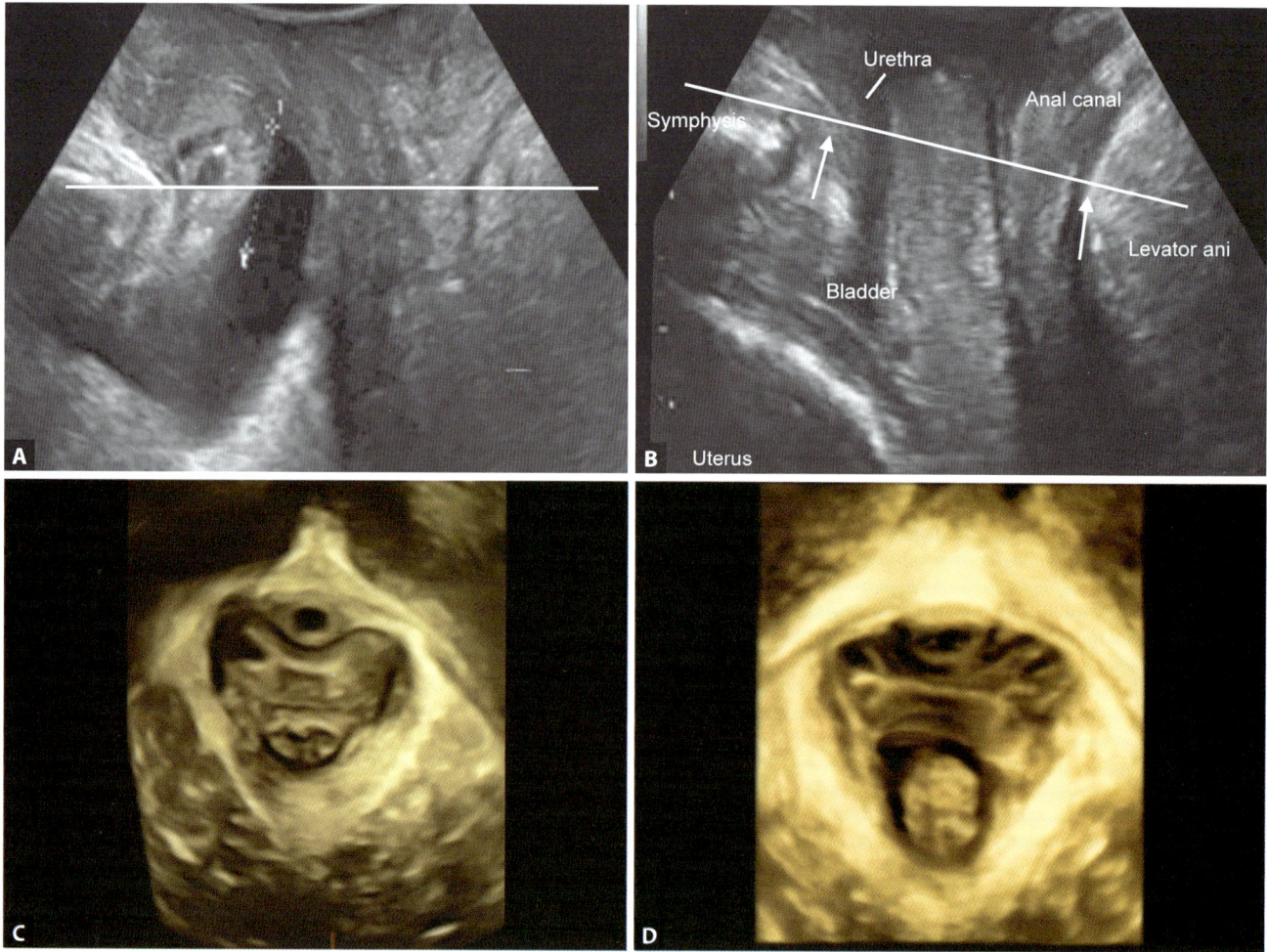

Figs. 6A to D: Midsagittal plane of the pelvic floor, showing the reference line—line of minimal hiatal diameter, with difference in the position of the line in both images: (A) It is seen during Valsalva; (B) It is seen on levator coactivation; (C and D) The same instances on axial image of 3D ultrasound of pelvic floor showing decrease in the AP diameter on Valsalva.

Larger hiatal area than this indicates risk of prolapse:
- Mild overdistention (25–29.9 cm^2)
- Moderate overdistention (30–34.9 cm^2)
- Marked overdistention (35–39.9 cm^2)
- Severe overdistention (40+ cm^2)

Posterior compartment assessment:
- Rectoenterocele **(Fig. 10)**
- Enterocele
- Rectal prolapse
- Rectal intussusception

Rectoceles are associated with intact but abnormally distensible rectovaginal septum. These commonly present as incomplete bowel emptying, futile straining for stool, and rectal prolapse.

Rectal Intussusception

In the case of RI, the full thickness of the rectal wall invaginates into the anal canal.[39] This may produce a bulge on the posterior vaginal wall, easily mistaken for rectocele or enterocele; and it presents as obstructed defecation.[39,40]

It is more common in patients with a clinical diagnosis of rectocele or enterocele.[40] This condition may be detected by 2D or 3D TUS with satisfactory levels of sensitivity and specificity.[41]

Bilateral levator ani atrophy results in prolapse of all the three compartments.

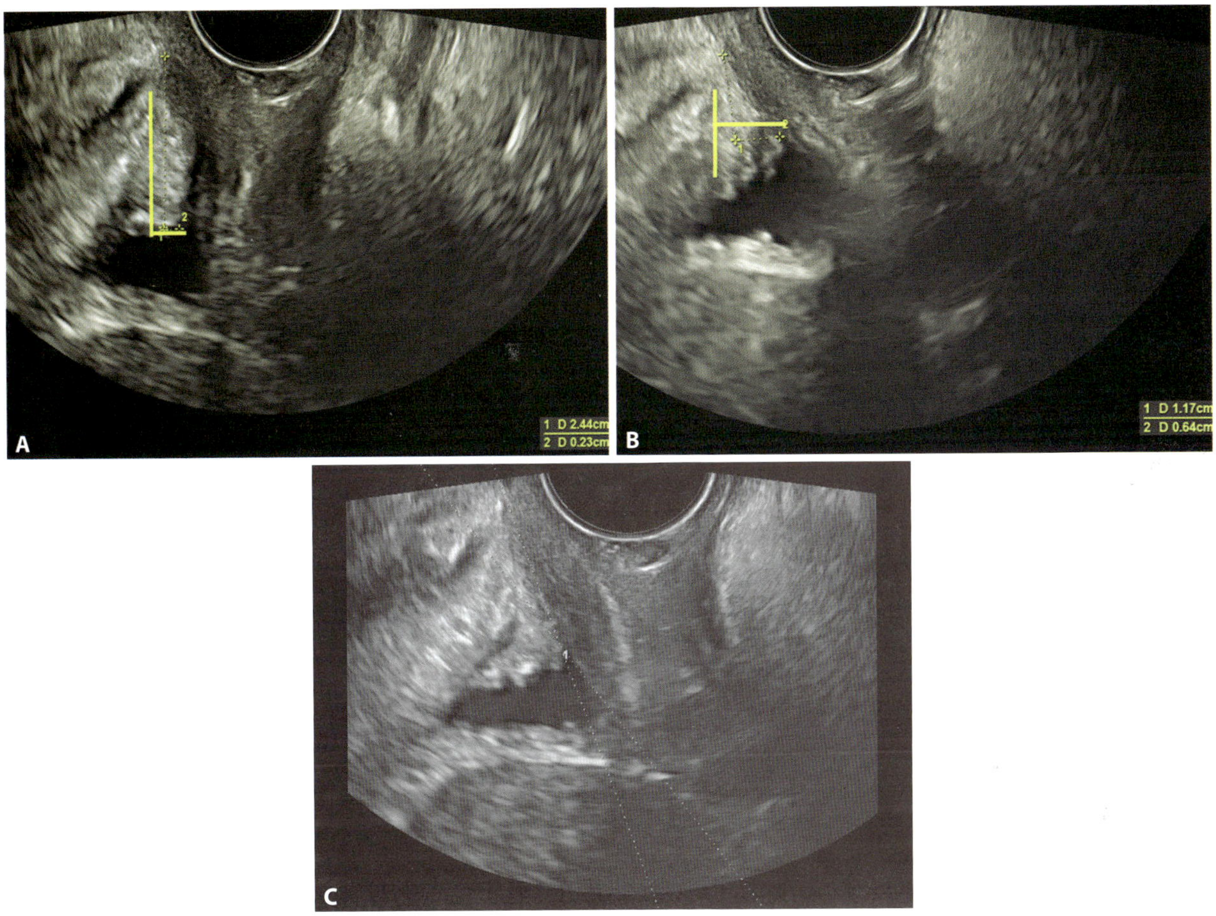

Figs. 7A to C: (A and B) Vertical distance of bladder neck from lower margin of symphysis pubis and transverse line showing AP distance of the vesicourethral junction from this line at rest and on Valsalva respectively; (C) Midsagittal plane of bladder neck on B-mode ultrasound showing measurement of posterior urethrovesical angle.

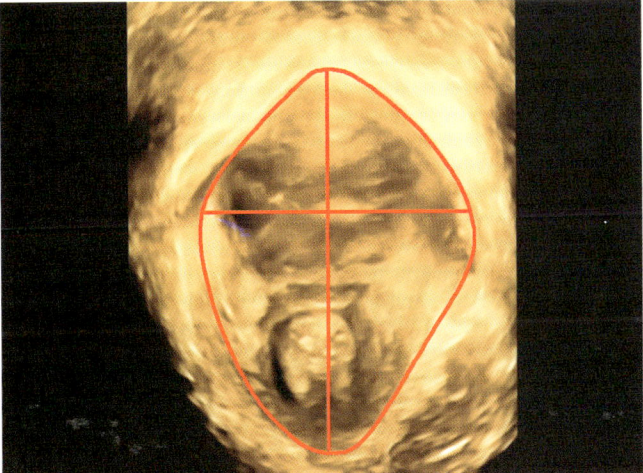

Fig. 8: 3D ultrasound, multiplanar image of the axial section of the pelvic floor. AP and transverse diameter of the pelvic floor and circumference are measured.

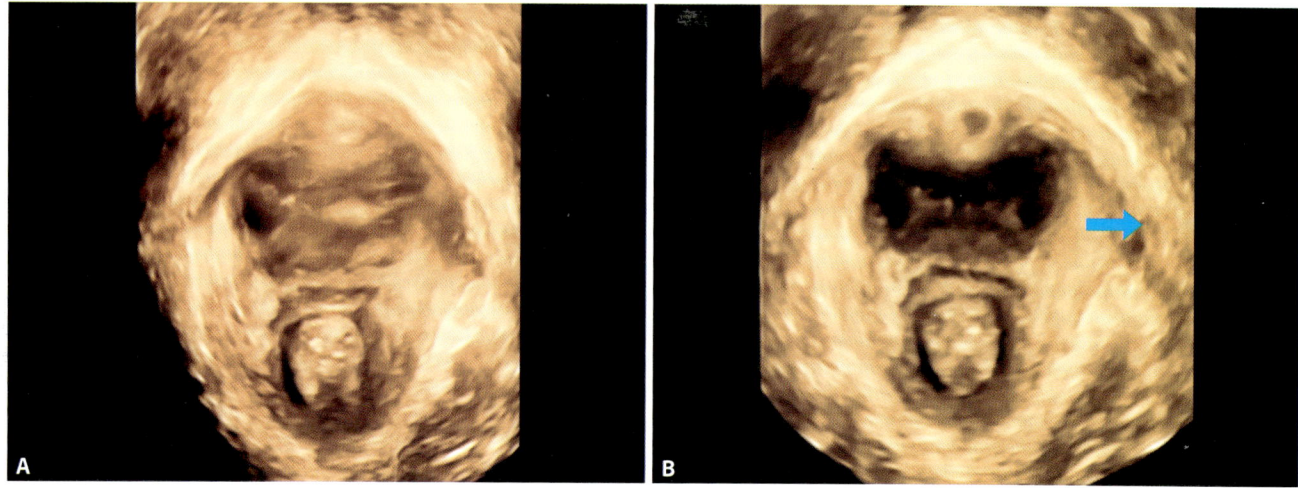

Figs. 9A and B: (A) Normal 3D rendered image of the axial section of the pelvic floor; (B) In a similar section, blue arrow showing avulsion of levator ani.

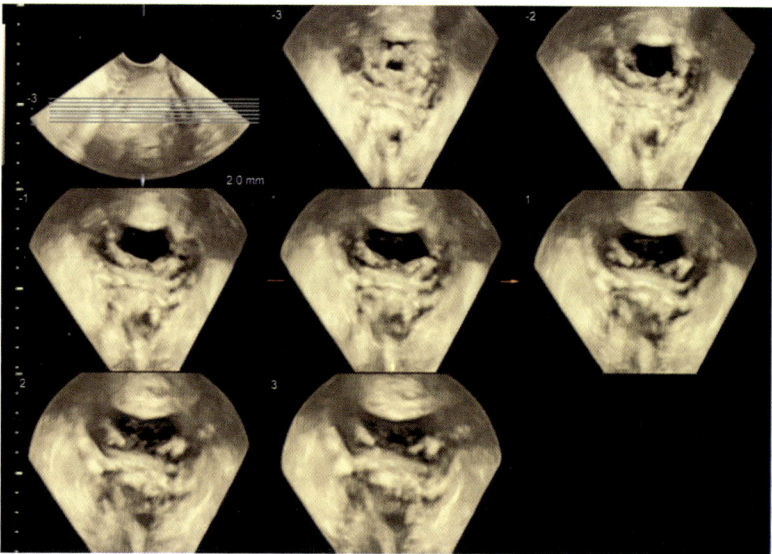

Fig. 10: 3D ultrasound image of the pelvic floor showing large urethral meatus and bladder neck with bulging bowel loops in the vagina suggestive of funneling of the bladder neck and enterocele.

CONCLUSION

Availability of pelvic floor ultrasound has revolutionized the understanding of morphological anomalies of levator ani. The cause of these abnormalities is now understood to be injury to the muscles of pelvic floor—traumatic avulsion of the muscles. Levator ani trauma leads to anterior and middle compartment prolapse.[42] Abnormal puborectalis may lead to fecal incontinence.[43] If avulsion is bilateral, it may lead to effect on sexual function. Ultrasound may be proposed as the initial examination of choice. Ultrasound may be used for assessment of bladder neck mobility before anti-incontinence procedures.

Correlation with symptoms and guide to treatment:[44]
- *Recurrent lower urinary tract infections:* Atrophied endopelvic fascia and increased residual urine, cystocele/overcorrection of urethra; may also be associated with bladder or urethral diverticuli, intravesical calculi, foreign body or abnormally located intrauterine device.

- *Urgency and frequency of urine:* Periurethral or intravesical masses, bladder and urethral diverticuli, anterior uterine fibroids, and funneling of proximal urethra.
- *Dysuria and dyspareunia:* UD, periurethral masses, and migrating intrauterine contraceptive device
- *Urge:* Thick bladder wall
- *SUI:* Hypermobile urethra, reduced or absent pelvic floor activity, cystocele, and funneling.

REFERENCES

1. Shek KL, Deitz HP. Intrapartum risk factors of levator trauma. BJOG. 2006;26:710-6.
2. Dietz HP, Steensma AB, Hastings R. Three dimensional ultrasound imaging of pelvic floor: The effect of parturition on paravaginal support structures. Ultrasound Obstet Gynecol. 2003;21:589-95.
3. Dietz HP. Ultrasound imaging of the pelvic floor: Part II: three-dimensional or volume imaging. Ultrasound Obstet Gynecol. 2004;23:615-25.
4. Youssef A, Montaguti E, Sanlorenzo O, Cariello L, Salsi G, Morganelli G, et al. Reliability of new three-dimensional ultrasound technique for pelvic hiatal area measurement. Ultrasound Obstet Gynecol. 2016;47(5):629-35.
5. Deitz H, Shek KL. Tomographic ultrasound imaging of the pelvic floor: Which level matters most? Ultrasound Obstet Gynecol. 2009;33(6):698-703.
6. Kruger JA, Heap SW, Murphy BA, Dietz HP. Pelvic floor function in nulliparous women using three-dimensional ultrasound and magnetic resonance imaging. Obstet Gynecol. 2008;111(3):631-8.
7. Weinstein MM, Jung SA, Pretorius DH, Nager CW, den Boer DJ, Mittal RK. The reliability of puborectalis muscle measurement with 3-dimensional ultrasound imaging. Am J Obstet Gynecol. 2007;197(1):68.e1-e6.
8. Santoro GA, Wieczorek AP, Dietz HP, Mellgren A, Sultan AH, Shobeiri SA, et al. State of the art: An integrated approach to pelvic floor ultrasonography. Ultrasound Obstet Gynecol. 2011;37(4):381-96.
9. Fitzgerald MP, Jaffar J, Brubaker L. Risk factors for an elevated postvoid residual urine volume in women with symptoms of urinary urgency, frequency, and urge incontinence. Int Urogynecol J Pelvic Floor Dysfunct. 2001;12(4):237-9.
10. Dietz HP. Pelvic floor ultrasound: A review. Am J Obstet Gynecol. 2010;202(4):321-34.
11. Tunn R, Schaer G, Peschers U, Bader W, Gauruder A, Hanzal E, et al. Updated recommendations on ultrasonography in urogynecology. Int Urogynecol J Pelvic Floor Dysfunct. 2005;16(3):236-41.
12. Weber AM, Abrams P, Brubaker L, Cundiff G, Davis G, Dmochowski RR, et al. The standardization of terminology for researchers in female pelvic floor disorders. Int Urogynecol J Pelvic floor Dysfunct. 2001;12(3):178-86.
13. Khullar V, Cardozo LD, Salvatore S, Hill S. Ultrasound: A noninvasive screening test for detrusor instability. Br J Obstet Gynecol. 1996;103(9):904-8.
14. Schaer GN, Koechli OR, Schuessler B, Haller U. Perineal ultrasound for evaluating the bladder neck in urinary stress incontinence. Obstet Gynecol. 1995;85(2):220-4.
15. Schaer G, Koelbl H, Voigt R, Merz E, Anthuber C, Niemeyer R, et al. Recommendations of the German association of Urogynecology on functional sonography of the lower female urinary tract. Int Urogynecol J Pelvic floor Dysfunct. 1996;7(2):105-8.
16. Khullar V, Salvatore S, Cardozo L, Bourne TH, Abbott D, Kekkeher C. A novel technique for measuring bladder wall thickness in women using transvaginal ultrasound. Ultrasound Obstet Gynecol. 1994;4(3):220-3.
17. Tunn R, Petri E. Introital and transvaginal ultrasound as the main tool in the assessment of urogenital and pelvic floor dysfunction: An imaging panel and practical approach. Ultrasound Obstet Gynecol. 2003;22(2):205-13.
18. Peschers UM, Vodušek DB, Fanger G, Schaer GN, De Lancey JO, Schuessler B. Pelvic muscle activity in nulliparous volunteers. Neurourol Urodyn. 2001;20(3):269-75.
19. Miller JM, Perucchini D, Carchidi LT, DeLancey JO, Ashton-Miller J. Pelvic floor muscle contraction during a cough and decreased vesical neck mobility. Obstet Gynecol. 2001;97(2):255-60.
20. Tunn R, Paris S, Fischer W, Hamm B, Kuchinke J. Static magnetic resonance imaging of the pelvic floor muscle morphology in women with stress urinary incontinence and pelvic prolapse. Neurourol Urodyn. 1998;17:579-89.
21. Medina CA, Costantini E, Petri E, Mourad S, Singla A, Rodríguez-Colorado S, et al. Evaluation and surgery for stress urinary incontinence: A FIGO working group report. Neurourol Urodyn. 2017;36(2):518-28.
22. Tseng LH, Liang CC, Chang YL, Lee SJ, Lloyd LK, Chen CK. et al. Postvoid residual urine in women with stress incontinence. Neurourol Urodyn. 2008;27(1):48-51.
23. Lekskulchai O, Dietz HP. Detrusor wall thickness as a test for detrusor overactivity in women. Ultrasound Obstet Gynecol. 2008;32(4):535-9.
24. Huang WC, Yang JM, Yang YC, Yang SH. Ultrasonographic characteristics and cystoscopic correlates of bladder wall invasion by endophytic cervical cancer. Ultrasound Obstet Gynecol. 2006;27(6):680-6.
25. El-Nashar SA, Bacon MM, Kim-Fine S, Weaver AL, Gebhart JB, Klingele CJ. Incidence of female urethral diverticulum: A population-based analysis and literature review. Int Urogynecol J. 2014;25(1):73-9.
26. Burrows LJ, Howden NL, Meyn L, Weber AM. Surgical procedures for urethral diverticula in women in the United States, 1979–1997. Int Urogynecol J Pelvic Floor Dysfunct. 2005;16(2):158-61.

27. Aldridge CW Jr, Beaton JH, Nanzig RP. A review of office urethroscopy and cystometry. Am J Obstet Gynecol. 1978;131(4):432-7.
28. Crescenze IM, Goldman HB. Femal urethral diverticulum: Current diagnosis and management. Curr Urol Rep. 2015;16(10):71.
29. Gerrard ER Jr, Lloyd LK, Kubricht WS, Kolettis PN. Transvaginal ultrasound for the diagnosis of urethral diverticulum. J Urol. 2003;169(4):1395-7.
30. Huang WC, Yang JM. Bladder neck funneling on ultrasound cystourethrography in primary stress urinary incontinence: A sign associated with urethral hypermobility and intrinsic sphincter deficiency. Urology. 2003;61(5):936-1.
31. Digesu GA, Khullar V, Cardozo L, Salvatore S. The open bladder neck: A significant finding? Int Urogynecol J Pelvic Floor Dysfunct. 2004;15(5):336-9.
32. Dietz HP. Ultrasound imaging of the pelvic floor. Part I: Two-dimensional aspects. Ultrasound Obstet Gynecol. 2004;23:80-92.
33. Dietz HP, Steensma AB, Vancaillie TG. Levator function in nulliparous women. Int Urogynecol J Pelvic Floor Dysfunct. 2003;14(1): 24-6.
34. DeLancy JOL. Structural support of the urethra as it relates to stress urinary incontinence: The hammock hypothesis. Am J Obstet Gynecol. 1994;170:1713-20.
35. DeLancy JO. Stress urinary incontinence. Where are we now, where should we go? Am J Obstet Gynecol. 1996;175(2):311-9.
36. Dietz HP, Wilson PD, Clarke B. The use of perineal ultrasound to quantify levator activity and teach pelvic floor muscle exercises. Int Urogynecol J Pelvic floor Dysfunct. 2001;12(3):166-8.
37. Abrams P, Cardozo L, Fall M, Griffiths D, Rosier P, Ulmsten U, et al.; Standardisation Sub-Committee of the International Continence Society. The standardization of terminology of lower urinary tract function: Report from the standardisation Sub-committee of the International Continence Society. Urology. 2003;61(1):37-49.
38. Delancey JO. Anatomy. In: Cardozo L, Staskin D (Eds). Textbook of Female Urology and Urogynaecology. London, UK: Isis Medical Media; 2001. pp. 112-24.
39. Rodrigo N, Shek KL, Dietz HP. Rectal intussusception is associated with abnormal levator ani muscle structure and morphometry. Tech Coloproctol. 2011;15(1):39-43.
40. Guzman Rojas R, Kamisan Atan I, Shek KL, Dietz HP. The prevalence of abnormal posterior compartment anatomy and its association with obstructed defecation symptoms in urogynecological patients. Int Urogynecol J. 2016;27(6):939-44.
41. Beer-Gabel M, Carter D. Comparison of dynamic trans-perineal ultrasound and defecography for the evaluation of pelvic floor disorders. Int J Colorectal Dis. 2015;30:835-41.
42. Deitz H, Simpson JM. Levator trauma is associated with pelvic organ prolapse. BJOG. 2008;115:979-84.
43. Chantarasorn V, Shek KL, Dietz HP. Sonographic detection of puborectalis muscle avulsion is not associated with anal incontinence. Aust N Z J Obstet Gynaecol. 2011;51(2):130-5.
44. Khurana A. Ultrasound in urogynecology. In: Kurjak A, Chervenak F (Eds). Donald School Textbook of Ultrasound in Obstetrics and Gynecology, 4th edition. New Delhi: Jaypee Brothers Medical Publishers (P) Ltd.; 2017.

Index

Page numbers followed by *b* refer to box, *f* refer to figure, *fc* refer to flowchart, and *t* refer to table

A

Abdominal wall defects 109
Achondrogenesis 109
Acrania 107
Adenocarcinoma 60
Adenomyoma 22
    focal 22, 24*f*
Adenomyosis 22
    focal 22
    signs of 8*f*
Adhesions 9
Adnexa, routine evaluation of 8
Adnexal lesions 61
    malignant 62*b*
Adnexal signs 110
Allis forceps 94
Alobar holoprosencephaly 107
Amenorrhea, primary 63
American Society for Reproductive Medicine 86
Amniotic
    cavity 103, 104
    membrane 106
    sac 103*f*, 104, 109*f*
Anal canal 115
Androblastomas 63
Anechoic cystic lesion 41*f*
Anechoic myometrial cysts 22
Anesthesia 94
Anovulation 86
Anterior compartment assessment 68
Anterior wall defect 108
Anti-Müllerian hormone 71, 88
Antral follicle count 71, 72, 72*f*, 74, 75, 86, 88, 88*f*
Anus 116*f*
Arteriovenous shunts 65*f*
Artery 5
Asepsis 99

B

Beta-human chorionic gonadotropin 102
Bladder 115
    base 69
    descent of 16*f*
    dome 69
    extra-abdominal 69
    neck 122*f*
        funneling of 16, 117, 118, 122*f*
        mobility 15, 117, 118
        vertical distance of 121*f*
    neurogenic 117
    tumors 15, 117, 118
    volume 15, 117
        measurement 117
    wall thickness 15, 117, 118
Bleeding 37
Body mass index 73-7, 88
Body stalk abnormalities 108
Border scar out 35
Bowel
    endometriosis 9*f*
        typical 69*f*
        interrupting anterior muscularis of 9*f*
Brain vesicles 103
Bulging bowel loops 122*f*

C

Calvarium 104
Cannula, removal of 100*f*
Carcinoma
    cervical 59
    endometrial 58, 59
Caudal regression syndrome 108
Cerebellum 104
Cervical
    assessment 42, 42*f*
        difficulties for 43
        methods of 42
    canal 40*f*, 41*f*
    fibroid 41*f*, 42
    funneling 44*f*
    incompetence 42
    insufficiency 43
    length 42, 43
        assessment of 42, 42*fc*, 43
        elasticity 42
        measurement 43*f*
    malignancy 14, 42
    mass 61*f*
    morphology 39
    pathologies, benign 39
    septa 14
Cervix 11, 14, 17, 39, 40*f*, 41, 41*f*, 60*f*
    anatomy of 39*f*
    assessment of 39, 42*t*
    malignancy of 57
    serial measurements of 43
Cesarean section 25, 34*f*
    scar 34, 111
Chocolate cyst 9*f*
Chorioangioma 112, 112*f*
Choriocarcinoma 62, 64
Chorionic tissue, tumors of 112
Choroid plexus 104, 104*f*
Coagulopathy 23
Cogwheel appearance 56*f*
Color Comet sign 102
Color Doppler 11, 27*f*, 73*f*, 77*f*, 83*f*
Contraception, hormonal 36
Copper-T 36
Cornual fibroid 26*f*
Corpus luteal
    Doppler parameters 84*t*
    flow 84
Corpus luteum 85, 98*f*, 102, 110
    formation of 83
Crown-rump length 105
Current ovum retrieval technique 94*f*
Cusco's speculum 99
Cystic degeneration 26*f*
Cystic endometrial hyperplasia 30*f*
Cystic lesion 8
Cystocele 15, 117, 119
Cystourethrocele 15, 117
Cytotrophoblast 64

D

Deep-infiltrating endometriosis 8, 67, 68
    scan technique for 8

Detrusor
   overactivity 118
   wall thickness 118
Diethylstilbestrol exposure 45
Doppler 10, 22, 76, 79
   assessment essential 77
   ultrasound study 5
Double-decidual ring sign 103
Double-lumen suction catheter 96*f*
Douglas pouch 4, 8, 9
Dysgerminoma 62, 63
Dysmenorrhea 37
Dysmorphic uterus 19
Dyspareunia 37
Dysuria, persistent 114

E

Early pregnancy, abnormal 102
Echogenicity, heterogeneous 65*f*
Ectopic pregnancy 110, 112*f*
Edema 28
Elective cervical cerclage 44
Embryo transfer 99, 99*f*, 100*f*
   cannula 41
   cycles 77
   suboptimal 100
   technique 99*b*
   ultrasound-guided 101
Embryonic pole 103*f*
Endometrial cavity 26*f*, 30*f*, 111*f*
Endometrial Doppler 6
Endometrial fibroid 29, 32*f*
Endometrial hyperplasia 28, 29, 30*f*
   differential diagnosis of 31*fc*
Endometrial lesions
   benign 28
   inflammatory 28*fc*
Endometrial lips, asymmetrical thickness of 102*f*
Endometrial neoplastic lesions 29
   differential diagnosis of 31*fc*
Endometrial pathologies 10, 28
Endometrial polyp 10*f*, 29, 32*f*, 33*t*, 59
Endometrial vascularity 7*f*, 79, 80*t*
Endometriosis 67, 67*fc*
   cervical deep-infiltrating 68
   diagnosis of 67
   superficial 69, 69*f*
   ultrasound evaluation for 8*b*
   vaginal 14
Endometriotic lesions 69
Endometriotic patch 67
Endometritis
   acute 28, 29*f*
   chronic 28, 29*f*, 84

Endometrium 6, 7*f*, 28, 57, 78, 79, 80*f*, 81*f*, 81*t*, 83
   Doppler features of 79
   Grade
     A 78*f*
     B 79*f*
     C 79*f*
   heterogeneous 22
   multilayered 81*f*
   question mark sign of 8, 22
   thickened 29*f*, 58*f*
   thin 29*f*
Enterocele 15, 117, 120, 122*f*
Epithelioid trophoblastic tumor 64
Estrogen 28
European Society of Human Reproduction and Embryology 86
Exomphalos 109

F

Fallopian tube 28, 110
   malignancy of 63
Falx 104
Fecal incontinence 114
Female pelvis, anatomy of 115*f*
Fetal abnormalities 104, 106
Fetal pole 104, 106
Fibroblasts 63
Fibroids 22, 33*t*, 110
   degenerated 26*f*
   polyps 33
Foley's bulb 12*f*
Follicle
   arrangement of 88
   aspiration equipment 96*f*
   gains 76
   lumen 81
   number per ovary 72, 86, 93
   transvesical aspiration of 94
   volume of 78
   wall 97*f*
Follicle-stimulating hormone 71, 76, 88
Follicular volume 77
Free fluid, differential diagnosis of 56*fc*
Frozen embryo transfer 74
Functional uterocervical length 99*f*
Fusion arrest 17

G

Gastroschisis 109
Gel vaginosonography 14
General cystic pattern 88
Generalized polycystic pattern 89*f*

Genitourinary prolapse 114
Germ cell tumors 62, 63
   malignant 63
Gestational sac 102-105, 105*f*, 109, 110, 111*f*
   abnormal 106
Gestational trophoblastic neoplasia 64
Glandular endometrial hyperplasia 30*f*
Glass body rendering 63*f*
Gonadoblastoma, gonadal dysgenesis of 63
Gonadotropin hormone-releasing hormone antagonist 71
Good quality
   endometrium 81
   follicle 81
Granulosa cell tumor 62, 63
Ground-glass echogenicity 8, 9*f*
Growth pattern, abnormal 104
Gynecological malignancy 57
   ultrasound in 57

H

Healthy scar 34*f*
Heart defects, major 109
Hematoma 15, 117
   subchorionic 107*f*
Hemivertebrae 109
Heterogeneity
   causes of 8
   extent of 8
Hiatus ballooning 117
Holoprosencephaly 107, 109*f*
Homogeneous echo structure 36
Hormonal implications 90
Hormones 28
Human chorionic gonadotropin 74, 80, 85, 105
Human papilloma virus 59
Human placental lactogen 64
Hydropic villi invade 64
Hydrosalpinx 64*f*, 98*f*
   acutely inflamed 56*f*
Hyperandrogenism 86
Hyperdense stroma 89
Hyperechoic flecks 9, 69*f*
Hyperechoic stroma 89
Hyperemia 28
Hyperplasia 23
   endometrial 28, 29, 30*f*
Hypoechoic lesion 68, 69*f*
Hypoechoic nodules 69*f*
Hypophosphatasia 109
Hystero-contrast sonography 11, 12, 13*f*

I

Iliac vessels, external 4*f*
Immature teratomas 62
In vitro fertilization 72, 74, 75, 99
    cycle 74, 74*fc*, 75*fc*, 77
    procedures 94
Inflammation, hyperemia of acute 28
Injury, endometrial 84
Insulin 90
    like growth factor 90
International Deep Endometriosis
        Analysis 68
International Federation of Gynecology
        and Obstetrics 22, 41, 117
Intervening muscle wall, absorption of 17
Intralesional vascularity 25*f*
Intramural fibroid 25*f*
    large 26*f*
Intrauterine contraceptive device 34, 36
    in situ 37*f*
Intrauterine insemination 74, 75, 75*fc*
    cannula 41
    cycle 74, 74*fc*
Intrauterine pregnancy
    confirmation of 102
    diagnostic of 102
Introital ultrasound 117
Invasive mole 64
Isthmocele 34, 34*f*, 36*f*, 37
    causes of 34*f*

K

Kissing ovaries 9
Kyphoscoliosis 108

L

Leiomyoma 22
Levator ani
    atrophy, bilateral 120
    avulsion of 122*f*
    trauma 122
Levator coactivation 119, 120*f*
Levator hiatus 114
Leydig cell 63
    tumor 62, 63
Limb abnormalities, major 107
Localized myometrial lesions,
        classification of 24*f*
Lower uterine segment
    continuous contour of 36
    echoing structure of 35
    V shape of 35
Lumen polyps 40*f*
Luteal phase
    abnormal 85, 85*fc*
    defect 84
    normal 85, 85*fc*
    scan 83
Luteal support 85
Luteinizing hormone 74, 76, 85, 88

M

Magnetic resonance imaging 17, 70
Malignancy 57, 58*f*, 59*f*
    index, risk of 61
    endometrial 29, 33, 33*f*, 58*f*
Mass, malignant 59*f*
Mature follicle 76*f*
    aspiration of 94
Maximum levator thickness 117
Mayer-Rokitansky-Küster-Hauser
        syndrome 21
Membranes
    preterm premature rupture of 44
    rupture of 45
Mesencephalon 103
Metastatic ovarian tumor 62, 63, 63*f*
Mirena 36
Mucinous epithelial tumors 62
Müllerian ducts
    abnormalities 17
    formation of 17
    fusion of 17
Multiloculated solid mass 62*f*
Multiple gestations,
        early detection of 102, 113
Multiple regression analysis 44
Multiple subendometrial fibroids 32*f*
Myometrial cysts 8*f*
Myometrial homogeneity 8
Myometrial lesions 22, 22*fc*
Myometrial thickness 36*f*
Myometrial vascularity 25, 27*f*
Myometrium 37, 57
    asymmetrical thickening of 8*f*
    continuity of 35
    thickened 23*f*

N

Nabothian cyst 41, 41*f*
Negative predictive value 43, 61
Neoplastic lesions 29
Niche depth, measurement of 36

O

Omphalocele 104*f*, 109
Omphalomesenteric duct 103
Oocytes 77
    retrieval 94, 95*fc*
        complications of 98*fc*
Organ 39
Orthogonal diameter 6*f*, 107*f*
    measurement 118*f*
Ovarian area 90
    measurement of 90*f*
Ovarian artery perfusion 83
Ovarian beak sign 53*f*
Ovarian calcinosis 53*f*
Ovarian hyperstimulation syndrome 74
Ovarian malignancies 57
Ovarian rim sign 53*f*
Ovarian steroids 28
Ovarian stromal flow 5, 72, 73*f*
    measurement of 72
Ovarian stromal peak systolic velocity 72
Ovarian tumors, malignant 61
Ovarian volume 71, 72, 73*f*, 74*t*,
    75, 86, 90, 91, 93
Ovary 2*f*, 5*f*, 6*f*, 12*f*, 72*f*, 90*f*, 91*f*, 98, 98*f*
    transverse section of 4*f*
Overactive bladder syndrome 117
Ovulation induction 74*fc*, 74*t*
Ovulatory dysfunction 23
Ovum pickup 96*f*, 97*f*, 98
    needle 96*f*

P

Paraovarian cyst 53*f*
Peak systolic velocity 72, 74-76, 83, 102
Pedunculated ovarian fibroma 54*f*
Pedunculated uterine fibroid 54*f*
Pelvic floor 15, 116*f*, 122*f*
    anatomy of 114
    axial section of 121*f*
    imaging 115*fc*
    midsagittal plane of 120*f*
Pelvic inflammatory disease 28, 52
Pelvic organs
    orientation of 2
    prolapse 117
    transabdominal scan of 2
Pelvic outlet, transverse
        diameter of 16, 16*f*
Pelvic pain, chronic 37
Pelvis 56*fc*
    extraovarian lesions of 52, 52*fc*
    longitudinal section of 2*f*
    transverse section of 2*f*, 4*f*
Perifollicular flow 6, 7*f*
    index 77
Perifollicular vascularization index 77
Perineal region, basic anatomy of 115*f*

Perineum, axial section of 116*f*
Peripheral hyperechoic ring 22
Peripheral polycystic pattern 89*f*
Peripheral vascularity 25*f*, 112*f*
Peritoneal cavity 35*f*
Peritoneal inclusion cyst 53*f*
Peritoneal surface 67
Phantom perineum 15*f*
Placental site trophoblastic tumor 64
Polycystic ovarian syndrome 92, 92*fc*
    diagnosis of 86, 90
Polycystic ovary 86, 87, 87*f*, 88, 88*f*, 89, 89*f*, 90, 91*t*
    dense hyperechoic stroma of 90*f*
Polyp 22, 59*f*
    cervical 14, 40-42
Positive predictive value 43, 61
Posterior compartment assessment 68
Pregnancy 104, 110, 112
    angular 109, 111*f*
    assessment, Early 105*fc*
    cervical 110
        ectopic 42
    cornual 110, 111
    ectopic 112*f*
    growth of 103
    interstitial 110, 111
    intrauterine 102
    losses, repeated mid-trimester 45
    normal early 102
    ovarian ectopic 110, 112*f*
    scar 110
    viability of 103
Preovulatory follicle 81*t*
Preovulatory scan 81
Preterm delivery, high-risk population for 44
Preterm labor, symptoms of 44
Pretrigger follicle 81
Probe
    position of 15*f*
    pressure, tenderness on 9, 22
Progesterone 28
Prosencephalon 103
Pseudogestational sac 111, 111*f*
Puborectalis 114
Pubourethral angle 16
Pulsatility index 83, 85, 91
Pulse Doppler 73*f*, 83*f*
Pulse repetition frequency 1, 5, 61, 72, 77
Puncture hydrosalpinx 97

R

Recombinant follicle-stimulating hormone 74
Rectal intussusception 15, 117, 120
Rectal prolapse 120
Rectocele 15, 117
Rectoenterocele 120
Rectosigmoid deep-infiltrating endometriosis 68
Rectovaginal endometriotic patch 68*f*
Rectum 115
Recurrent urinary tract infection 114, 122
Residual myometrial thickness 35
Resistance index 6, 58, 72, 74, 75, 83-85
Retropubic hematoma 118
Rhombencephalon 103, 103*f*
Rosebush thorn sign 81

S

Saline-infusion
    salpingography 11, 12*f*, 13*f*
    sonohysterography procedure 10
Salpingitis, acute 55*f*
Sarcoma 57
Scar
    thickness 35
    volume 35
Sclerocystic ovaries 86
Secretory endometrium 84*f*
Segmental uterine 83
Septated fluid collection 56*f*
Serous epithelial tumors 62
Sertoli cells 63
Sex cord 62, 63
Single-feeder vessel 32*f*
Single-lumen ovum pickup needle 96*f*
Sirenomelia 108
Skeletal dysplasias, major 108
Skull, ossification of 104
Small antral follicles, granulosa cell of 88
Small uterine body 60*f*
Soft tissue adnexal band 4*f*
Sonography-based automated volume count 72, 77, 86, 88*f*, 92
Sonohysterography 10*f*, 33, 54
Spectral Doppler, sample volume of 5*f*
Spina bifida 109
Spinal defects, major 109
Spiral artery flow 84
Squamous cell carcinoma 60
Stress urinary incontinence 117
Stromal abundance 89, 90
Stromal tumors 62, 63
Stromal vessels 6*f*
Subendometrial fibroid 32*f*
Surgery, cervical 45
Symmetrical endometrial lips 111*f*
Symphysis pubis 115, 115*f*, 116*f*, 121*f*
Syncytiotrophoblast 64
Synechiae 28, 29*f*

T

Talipes equino varus 109
Tissue planes 60*f*
Transabdominal scan 2*f*
Translabial ultrasound 42
Transperineal scan 15, 15*f*, 115*f*
Transrectal scan 68
Transvaginal cervical assessment 43
Transvaginal oocyte retrieval 94
Transvaginal scan 2, 3, 3*f*, 4*f*, 5, 5*f*, 6*f*, 14, 68
    essentials of 3
Transvaginal sonography 8, 43
Transvaginal ultrasound 37, 42, 114
    transducer 96*f*
Triangular endometrial cavity 109
Tubal assessment 11
Tubal lesions
    classification of 54*fc*
    differential diagnosis of 54*fc*
Tubal malignancies 57, 63
Tubal patency, evaluation of 11*f*
Tuberculosis 28
Tubo-ovarian mass 55*f*
Tumor
    epithelial 61, 62
    extension 61*f*
    solid part of 64*f*
    vessels 57

U

Ultrasonography
    cervical 44
    dynamic 8
Ultrasound 11, 54, 57, 58, 63, 65, 67, 70, 76, 81, 86, 92, 94
    contrast 57
    diagnostic criteria 17
    parameters 73
    probe 115*f*
    purpose of 8
    transabdominal 114
    transperineal 42, 114, 115
    two-dimensional 92
Unicornuate hemiuterus 17
Unicornuate uterus 17, 18*f*
Unilocular cystic tumor 62*f*
Unilocular solid lesion 62*f*
Urethra 115, 116*f*
    hypermobility of 15
Urethral diverticula 15, 117, 118

Urethral hypermobility 118
Urethral meatus, large 122f
Urinary bladder 118f, 119f
Urinary incontinence 114
    complex 117
Urine analysis 114
Urogynecology 114
Uterine
    abnormalities 110
        congenital 17, 45
    artery 5f, 91
        Doppler 5
        flow waveform, high resistance 80f
    cavity 100f
    cornu 101f
    descent 16
    lesions 34
    malformation, accessory
        cavitated 21, 21f
    malignancies 57
    scar 34, 35f
    signs 109
    structures 36
    wall 5
Uterosacral deep-infiltrating
    endometriosis 68
Uterosacral ligament 68, 69f
    thickened 69f
Uterus 2f-4f, 10f, 12f, 17, 22, 30f, 115f
    agenesis of 17
    anteverted 9
    arcuate 19, 20f
    assessment of 22, 22fc
    asymmetrical enlargement of 22
    bicornuate 17, 20f, 111
    bicorporeal 17, 20f
    body, malignancies of 57
    complete septate 20f
    development of 17
    didelphys 20f
    duplication abnormalities of 19fc
    formation abnormalities of 18fc
    heterogenous solid lesion of 58f
    hypoplastic 19
    infantilis 19
    midsagittal section of 34f
    mobility of 8
    position of 8
    retroverted 9
    routine evaluation of 8
    sagittal section of 23f
    septate 19
    symmetrical enlargement of 22
    transverse section of 3f, 25f
    T-shaped 19, 21f

V

Vagina 14, 95, 99, 115
Vaginal carcinoma, primary 60
Vaginal cystic lesions 14
Vaginal deep-infiltrating
    endometriosis 68
Vaginal malignancy 57, 60
Vaginal septa 14
Vaginal wall 60f, 119
    thickening 68
Vaginosonography 39
Valsalva maneuver 119
Vault prolapse 119
Vesicourethral angle 16
Vesicourethral junction 121f
Vesicular mole 112, 113f
Vessels 5, 33, 58
    variable caliber of 57
Virtual organ computer-aided
    analysis 59, 72, 73f, 78f, 86, 87f, 91f, 92, 106
Vulval malignancies 57

Y

Yolk sac 103, 103f, 104, 106
    irregular 108f
    large 108f
    measurement 108f
    solid 108f
    thick walled 108f
    tiny 108f
    tumors 62